Printed in the United States of America

Chapter 3: Grammar - 61

Chapter 4: Vocabulary - 81

Chapter 5: Biology - 95

Chapter 6: Chemistry - 125

Chapter 7: Anatomy & Physiology - 163

Chapter 7: Physics - 231

Practice Test #1 - 249

Practice Test #2 - 321

Introduction

Congratulations on your decision to join the field of health care! Few other professions are so rewarding. By purchasing this book, you've already made the first step towards succeeding in your career; and the second step is to do well on the HESI A2. The Health Education Systems Incorporated Admission Assessment (HESI A2) will require you to demonstrate knowledge and competence of those subjects taught at the high school level. This book will help refresh you on all of those subjects, as well as provide you with some inside-information on how to do well on this test. Even if it's been years since you've graduated high school, studied, or taken a test – don't worry, you'll be ready!

ABOUT THE TEST

The HESI A2 is a multi-section, computer-based exam. There are eight academically-oriented sections which you may encounter on the exam:

Mathematics

The Mathematics section of the HESI A2 is relatively easy in comparison to other entrance tests since the list of tested concepts is more limited. However, you must be highly proficient in those areas. You will encounter questions testing you on addition, subtraction, multiplication, You will also need to have a proficient knowledge of roman numbers, calculating dosages, household measures, and conversions. The Math section of the exam is 50 minutes long and has 50 questions.

Reading

Covers: Ability to Read, Analyze, and Comprehend short text passages related to health and medicine. You will encounter 50 questions and have 60 minutes to complete the section. You will need to be able to identify the main idea, themes of the passage, make inferences, and interpret information from context clues in the passages.

Vocabulary

You will be tested on your knowledge of words, specifically, those relating to the health field (although not all questions will be). You will have 50 minutes to answer 50 questions.

Grammar

The grammar sections will test your knowledge of basic grammar, parts of speech, common grammatical errors, and other related concepts. This section is 50 minutes long and has 50 questions.

Biology

The biology section covers topics such as biology basics, cellular respiration, photosynthesis, metabolism, biological molecules, and cells. The level of knowledge required is through the high school level. Biology, like the other science related sections, can be one of the most difficult as there are only 25 questions, but the concepts covers a wide spectrum of required knowledge. You will have 25 minutes to complete this section.

Chemistry

The Chemistry section covers topics such as the periodic table, chemical equations, atomic structure, chemical bonding, nuclear chemistry and chemical reactions. You will have 25 minutes to answer 25 questions.

Anatomy & Physiology

The Anatomy & Physiology section (often simply called "A&P"), is likely one of the most challenging for many test-takers. This is because often students might have had limited, if any, previous exposure to quality anatomy and physiology education. There are only 25 questions in which you have 25 minutes to answer, however this section covers a very wide spectrum of body systems such as: muscular, skeletal, nervous, renal/urinary, reproductive, endocrine, circulatory, and respiratory systems.

Physics

Very few test-takers will actually have the physics section on their exam as this is almost always excluded by most colleges/institutions. Many students might not even realize that it is part of the test (until they read this of course). If you do encounter it, you will be tested on motion, gravity, rotation, friction, gravitation, energy, average speed, Newton's Laws of Motion, projectile motion, light, optics and acceleration. Even if you do have this section on your test, do not focus your efforts here, the other sciences and mathematics are typically much more important.

Other "Un-Scored" Sections

You may also encounter other, un-scored sections on the HESI A2 called "personally oriented" exams. These exams will not be used to evaluate your score. Instead, they are designed to help students better understand their strengths and weaknesses, learning styles and habits, and other traits of their personality.

SCORING

You cannot "pass" or "fail" the HESI A2. Your score is simply indicative of your current level of comprehension. However, each school has their own entrance requirements – some are higher than others. Be sure to check with the requirements of the institutions which you want to attend. Also, each institution has different requirements regarding the *sections* of the test which you'll take; make sure to check that you're taking the proper exam, before you spend all your time studying for a subject which you won't necessarily need.

HOW THIS BOOK WORKS

The subsequent chapters in this book are divided into those subjects covered on the HESI A2 exam. This book is not intended to "teach" or "re-teach" concepts – there is no way to cram all of that material into one book! Instead, we are going to help you recall all of the information which you've already learned. Even more importantly, we'll show you how to apply that knowledge. Each chapter includes an extensive review, with plenty of examples to make sure you understand the concepts.

Finally, you'll have 2 full practice tests at the end so you know for sure you are ready. With time, practice, and determination, you'll be well-prepared for test day.

Chapter 1: Mathematics

The math section of the HESI A2 test covers areas of applied math such as fractions, decimals, ratios, proportions, etc. We'll cover these subjects, and provide some additional strategies as well, within this chapter.

The Most Common Mistakes

People make mistakes all the time – but during a test, those mistakes can make the difference between an excellent score, or one which falls below the requirements. Watch out for these common mistakes that people make on the HESI A2:

- Answering with the wrong sign (positive / negative).

- Mixing up the Order of Operations.

- Misplacing a decimal.

- Not reading the question thoroughly (and therefore providing an answer that was not asked for.)

- Circling the wrong letter, or filling in wrong circle choice.

If you're thinking, "Those ideas are just common sense" – exactly! Most of the mistakes made on the HESI A2 are simple mistakes. Regardless, they still result in a wrong answer and the loss of a potential point.

Strategies for the Mathematics Section

1. **Go Back to the Basics**: First and foremost, practice your basic skills: sign changes, order of operations, simplifying fractions, and equation manipulation. These are the skills used most on the HESI A2, though they are applied in different contexts. Remember that when it comes right down to it, all math problems rely on the four basic skills of addition, subtraction, multiplication, and division. All that changes is the order in which they are used to solve a problem.

2. **Don't Rely on Mental Math**: Using mental math is great for eliminating answer choices, but ALWAYS WRITE IT DOWN! This cannot be stressed enough. Use whatever paper is provided; by writing and/or drawing out the problem, you are more likely to catch any mistakes. The act of writing things down forces you to organize your calculations, leading to an improvement in your HESI A2 score. Use your calculator to *check* your work.

3. **The Three-Times Rule**:

- **Step One – Read the question**: Write out the given information.

- **Step Two – Read the question**: Set up your equation(s) and solve.

- **Step Three – Read the question:** Make sure that your answer makes sense (is the amount too large or small, is the answer in the correct unit of measure, etc.).

4. **Make an Educated Guess**: Eliminate those answer choices which you are relatively sure are incorrect, and then guess from the remaining choices. Educated guessing is critical to increasing your score.

Math Concepts Tested on the HESI A2

You need to practice in order to score well on the test. To make the most out of your practice, use this guide to determine the areas for which you need more review. Most importantly, practice all areas under testing circumstances (a quiet area, a timed practice test, no looking up facts as you practice, etc.)

When reviewing, take your time and let your brain recall the necessary math. If you are taking the HESI A2, then you have already had course instruction in these areas. The examples given will "jog" your memory.

The next few pages will cover various math subjects (starting with the basics, but in no particular order), along with worked examples.

Positive & Negative Number Rules

Adding, multiplying, and dividing positive and negative numbers has predictable results. Knowing these can help determine if your answer is correct.

(+) + (-) = Solution has the sign of the larger number.

(-) + (-) = Negative number.

(-) * (-) = Positive number.

(-) * (+) = Negative number.

(-) / (-) = Positive number.

(-) / (+) = Negative number.

Examples:

Find the product of -10 and 47.

(-) * (+) = (-)

-10 * 47 = **-470**

What is the sum of -65 and -32?

(-) + (-) = (-)

-65 + -32 = **-97**

Is the product of -7 and 4 less than -7, between -7 and 4, or greater than 4?

(-) * (+) = (-)

-7 * 4 = -28, which is **less than -7**

What is the value of -16 divided by 2.5?

(-) / (+) = (-)

-16 / 2.5 = -6.4

Order of Operations

PEMDAS – **P**arentheses/**E**xponents/**M**ultiply/**D**ivide/**A**dd/**S**ubtract

This describes the order that math steps are done within a problem.

Perform the operations within parentheses first, and then any exponents. After those steps, perform all multiplication and division. (These are done from left to right, as they appear in the problem).

Finally, do all required addition and subtraction, also from left to right as they appear in the problem.

Examples:

1. Solve $(-(2)^2 - (4 + 7))$

   First, complete operations within parentheses:

   $(-(2)^2 - (11))$

   Second, calculate the value of exponential numbers:

   $(-(4) - (11))$

   Finally, do addition and subtraction:

   $(-(4) - (11)) = $ **-15**

2. Solve $(5)^2 \div 5 + 4 * 2$

   First, calculate the value of exponential numbers:

   $(25) \div 5 + 4 * 2$

   Second, calculate division and multiplication from left to right:

   $5 + 8$

   Finally, do addition and subtraction:

   $5 + 8 = $ **13**

3. Solve the expression $15 * (4 + 8) - 3^3$

First, complete operations within parentheses:

$15 * (12) - 3^3$

Second, calculate the value of exponential numbers:

$15 * (12) - 27$

Third, calculate division and multiplication from left to right:

$180 - 27$

Finally, do addition and subtraction from left to right:

$180 - 27 = \textbf{153}$

4. Solve the expression $(\frac{5}{2} * 4) + 23 - 4^2$

First, complete operations within parentheses:

$(10) + 23 - 4^2$

Second, calculate the value of exponential numbers:

$(10) + 23 - 16$

Finally, do addition and subtraction from left to right:

$(10) + 23 - 16$

$33 - 16 = \textbf{17}$

Greatest Common Factor (GCF)

The greatest common factor (GCF) of a group of numbers is the largest number that can evenly divide all of the numbers in the group. To find the GCF of a set, find all of the factors of each number in the set. A factor is a whole number that can be multiplied by another whole number to result in the original number. For example, the number 10 has four factors: 1, 2, 5, and 10. These are all of the whole numbers that can be multiplied by another whole number to equal the number 10.

When listing the factors of a number, remember to include 1 and the number itself.

The largest number that is a factor for each number in the set is the GCF.

Examples:

Find the GCF of 24 and 18.

Factors of 24: 1, 2, 3, 4, 6, 8, 12, 24

Factors of 18: 1, 2, 3, 6, 9, 18

The greatest common factor is **6**.

Find the GCF of 121 and 44.

Since these numbers are larger, it's easiest to start with the smaller number when listing factors.

Factors of 44: 1, 2, 4, 11, 22, 44

Now, it's not necessary to list all of the factors of 121. Instead, we can eliminate those factors of 44 which do not divide evenly into 121:

121 is not evenly divisible by 2, 4, 22, or 44 because it is an odd number. This leaves only 1 and 11 as common factors, so **11** is the GCF.

Greatest common factor problems can also appear as word problems. For example:

First aid kits are being assembled at a summer camp. A complete first aid kit requires bandages, sutures, and sterilizing swabs, and each of the kits must be identical to other kits. If the camp's total supplies include 52 bandages, 13 sutures, and 39 sterilizing swabs, how many complete first aid kits can be assembled without having any leftover materials?

This problem is asking for the greatest common factor of 52, 13, and 39. The first step is to find all of the factors of the smallest number, 13:

Factors of 13: 1, 13

13 is a prime number, meaning that its only factors are 1 and itself. Next, we check to see if 13 is also a factor of 39 and 52:

13 * 2 = 26
13 * 3 = 39
13 * 4 = 52

We can see that 39 and 52 are both multiples of 13. This means that **13 first aid kits** can be made without having any leftover materials.

Elena is making sundaes for her friends. She has 20 scoops of chocolate ice cream and 16 scoops of strawberry. If she wants to make identical sundaes and use all of her ice cream, how many sundaes can she make?

Arranging things into identical groups with no leftovers is always a tip that the problem calls for finding the greatest common factor. To find the GCF of 16 and 20, the first step is to factor both numbers:

Factors of 16: 1, 2, 4, 8, 16

Factors of 20: 1, 2, 4, 5, 10, 20

From these lists, we see that **4** is the GCF. Elena can make four sundaes, each with five scoops of chocolate ice cream and four scoops of strawberry. Any other combination would result in leftover ice cream or sundaes that are not identical.

Fractions

Adding and subtracting fractions requires a common denominator. The denominator is the number on the bottom of the fraction. The first step when adding or subtracting a set of fractions is the convert all of the fractions into numbers with common denominators. Once the denominators are the same, the numerators can be added or subtracted.

Find a common denominator for:

$$\frac{2}{3} - \frac{1}{5}$$

To find the common denominator, you can multiply each fraction by the number 1. With fractions, any number over itself is equivalent to 1. $\frac{5}{5}$, $\frac{12}{12}$, and $\frac{0.4}{0.4}$ are all equivalent to 1. By using these types of multipliers, you can change the denominators of fractions to be the same number for each fraction in the addition or subtraction problem. Just remember to also multiply the numerator. For example:

$$\frac{2}{3} - \frac{1}{5} = \frac{2}{3}\left(\frac{5}{5}\right) - \frac{1}{5}\left(\frac{3}{3}\right) = \frac{10}{15} - \frac{3}{15} = \frac{7}{15}.$$

To add mixed fractions, you can first add the whole numbers, and then the fractions.

$$2\frac{1}{4} + 1\frac{3}{4} = 3\frac{4}{4} = 4.$$

To subtract mixed fractions, convert to single fractions by multiplying the whole number by the denominator and adding the numerator. Then work as above.

$$2\frac{1}{4} - 1\frac{3}{4} = \frac{9}{4} - \frac{7}{4} = \frac{2}{4} = \frac{1}{2}.$$

To multiply fractions, convert any mixed fractions into single fractions and multiply the numerators together and the denominators together. Reduce to lowest terms if needed.

$$2\frac{1}{4} * 1\frac{3}{4} = \frac{9}{4} * \frac{7}{4} = \frac{63}{16} = 3\frac{15}{16}.$$

To divide fractions, first convert any mixed fractions into single fractions. Then invert the second fraction so that the denominator and numerator are switched. Last, multiply the fractions. Inverting a fraction changes multiplication to division.

$$2\frac{1}{4} \div 1\frac{3}{4} = \frac{9}{4} \div \frac{7}{4} = \frac{9}{4} * \frac{4}{7} = \frac{36}{28} = 1\frac{8}{28} = 1\frac{2}{7}.$$

Practice questions:

- $5\frac{2}{3} - 2\frac{1}{3} = ?$

  This is a mixed-fraction subtraction problem, so the first step is to subtract the whole numbers:

  $$5 - 2 = 3$$

  Then, subtract the fractions. They already have a common denominator, 3:

  $$\frac{2}{3} - \frac{1}{3} = \frac{1}{3}$$

  So the answer is $3\frac{1}{3}$.

- What is the product of $\frac{1}{12}$ and $\frac{6}{8}$?

  This is a fraction multiplication problem, so simply multiply the numerators together and the denominators together and then reduce:

  $$\frac{1}{12} * \frac{6}{8} = \frac{6}{96} = \frac{1}{16}$$

  Sometimes it's easier to reduce fractions before multiplying if you can:

  $$\frac{1}{12} * \frac{6}{8} = \frac{1}{12} * \frac{3}{4} = \frac{3}{48} = \frac{1}{16}$$

- Find $\frac{7}{8} \div \frac{1}{4}$.

  For a fraction division problem, invert the second fraction and then multiply and reduce:

  $$\frac{7}{8} \div \frac{1}{4} = \frac{7}{8} * \frac{4}{1} = \frac{28}{8} = \frac{7}{2}$$

- Find $2\frac{1}{3} - \frac{3}{2}$.

  This is a fraction subtraction problem with a mixed fraction, so the first step is to convert the mixed fraction to a normal fraction:

  $$2\frac{1}{3} = \frac{2*3}{3} + \frac{1}{3} = \frac{7}{3}$$

  Next, multiply each fraction by a factor of 1 to get a common denominator. How do you know which factor of 1 to use? Look at the other fraction and use the number found in that denominator:

  $$\frac{7}{3} * \frac{2}{2} = \frac{14}{6}$$

  $$\frac{3}{2} * \frac{3}{3} = \frac{9}{6}$$

  Now, subtract the fractions by subtracting the numerators:

  $$\frac{14}{6} - \frac{9}{6} = \frac{5}{6}$$

- Find the sum of $\frac{9}{16}, \frac{1}{2},$ and $\frac{7}{4}$.

  For this fraction addition problem, we need to find a common denominator. Notice that 2 and 4 are both factors of 16, so 16 can be the common denominator:

  $$\frac{1}{2} * \frac{8}{8} = \frac{8}{16}$$

  $$\frac{7}{4} * \frac{4}{4} = \frac{28}{16}$$

  $$\frac{9}{16} + \frac{8}{16} + \frac{28}{16} = \frac{45}{16}$$

- A recipe calls for $^1/_4$ of a cup of sugar. If 8 and a half batches of the recipe are needed, how many cups of sugar will be used?

  This is a fraction multiplication problem: $\frac{1}{4} * 8\frac{1}{2}$.

  First, we need to convert the mixed fraction into a full fraction:

  $$8\frac{1}{2} = \frac{8*2}{2} + \frac{1}{2} = \frac{17}{2}$$

  Now, multiply the fractions across the numerators and denominators, and then reduce:

  $$\frac{17}{2} * \frac{1}{4} = \frac{17}{8} \text{ cups of sugar.}$$

- Find the value of $\frac{2}{5} \div 1\frac{1}{5}$

  This is a fraction division problem, so the first step is to convert the mixed fraction to a full fraction:
  $$1\frac{1}{5} = \frac{5*1}{5} + \frac{1}{5} = \frac{6}{5}$$

  Now, divide the fractions. Remember to invert the second fraction, and then multiply normally:

  $$\frac{2}{5} * \frac{5}{6} = \frac{10}{30} = \frac{1}{3}$$

- Sabrina has $\frac{2}{3}$ of a can of red paint. Her friend Amos has $\frac{1}{6}$ of a can. How much red paint do they have combined?

  To add fractions, make sure that they have a common denominator. Since 3 is a factor of 6, 6 can be the common denominator:

  $$\frac{2}{3} * \frac{2}{2} = \frac{4}{6}$$

  Now, add the numerators:

  $$\frac{4}{6} + \frac{1}{6} = \frac{5}{6} \text{ of a can of red paint}$$

Percent, Part, & Whole

$$Percent = \frac{Part}{Whole}$$

A percent is the ratio of the part to the whole. Questions may give the part and the whole and ask for the percent, or give the percent and the whole and ask for the part, or give the part and the percent and ask for the value of the whole. The equation above can be rearranged to solve for any of these:

Percent = Part / Whole

Part = Whole * Percent

Whole = Part / Percent

Percents should always be expressed as a decimal number when solving. For example, if a problem uses the number 30%, change that number to 0.3 when solving. The percent sign (%) indicates that the decimal has been multiplied by 100, so divide the % by 100.

The word "of" usually indicates what the whole is in a problem. Remember that the part is smaller than the whole when the percent .

Examples:

Jim spent 30% of his paycheck at the fair. He spent $15 for a hat, $30 for a shirt, and $20 playing games. How much was his check? (Round to nearest dollar.)

Whole = Part / Percent

Whole = (15 + 30 + 20) / .30 = **$217.00**

45 is 15% of what number?

Whole = Part / Percent

Whole = 45 / 0.15

Whole = **300**

Greta and Max sell cable subscriptions. In a given month, Greta sells 45 subscriptions and Max sells 51. If 240 total subscriptions were sold in that month, what percent were not sold by Greta or Max?

24

Percent = Part / Whole

Percent = (51 + 45) / 240

Percent = 0.4, or 40%

This tells us that Greta and Max sold 40% of the subscriptions, so **60%** were sold by other employees.

What percent of 65 is 39?

Percent = Part / Whole

Percent = 39 / 65

Percent = 0.6, or 60%

Grant needs to score 75% on an exam. If the exam has 45 questions, at least how many does he need to answer correctly?

Part = Whole * Percent

Part = 45 * 0.75

Part = 33.75, so he needs to answer at least 34 questions correctly.

Emma scored 16% of her team's goals during a soccer season. If the team totaled 25 goals, how many did Emma score?

Part = Whole * Percent

Part = 25 * 0.16

Part = 4 goals

Percent Change

Percent Change = Amount of Change / Original Amount * 100.

Percent Increase = (New Amount – Original Amount) / Original Amount * 100.

Percent Decrease = (Original Amount – New Amount) / Original Amount * 100.

Amount Increase (or **Decrease**) = Original Price * Percent Markup (or Markdown).

Original Price = New Price / (Whole - Percent Markdown [or Markup]).

Example: A car that was originally priced at $8300 has been reduced to $6995. What percent has it been reduced?

(8300 – 6995) / 8300 * 100 = **15.72%**.

Ratios

A ratio tells how many of one thing exists in proportion to another thing. Unlike fractions, ratios do not give the amount of a part relative to a whole. To work with ratios, you can find the equivalent fraction. Do this by adding together the parts of the ratio to find the size of the whole.

Examples:

There are 90 voters in a room, and they are either Democrat or Republican. The ratio of Democrats to Republicans is 5:4. How many Republicans are there?

We know that there are 5 Democrats for every 4 Republicans in the room; that is what the ratio 5:4 means. To convert the ratio to fractions, add the parts together to find the whole:

5 + 4 = 9

Fraction of Democrats: $\frac{5}{9}$

Fraction of Republicans: $\frac{4}{9}$

If 4/9ths of the 90 voters are Republicans, then:

$\frac{4}{9} * 90 =$ **40 voters** are Republicans.

The ratio of students to teachers in a school is 15:1. If there are 38 teachers, how many students attend the school?

To solve this ratio problem, we do **not** need to find the whole number of people in the school, since we are solving for one part of the population (students) given the size of the other population (teachers). We know that:

For every 1 teacher, there are 15 students.

Therefore for 38 teachers, there are 38 * 15 students.

38 * 15 = **570 students** in the school.

A variety pack of cereal bars contains peanut butter flavor and chocolate flavor in a ratio of 3:2. If there are 20 bars total, how many of them are peanut butter flavored?

Convert the ratio to fractions:

$3 + 2 = 5$

Fraction of peanut butter flavor: $\frac{3}{5}$

If there are 20 bars total, then $\frac{3}{5} * 20 = $ **12 bars** are peanut butter flavored.

Proportions

There are two types of proportionality:

Direct Proportions: Two quantities that are directly proportional will increase or decrease in tandem. They change in the same direction.

Inverse Proportions: Two quantities which are inversely proportional will change in opposite directions. As one increases, the other will decrease.

To solve **direct** proportions, set up a fraction equation. For example:

A train traveling 120 miles takes 3 hours to get to its destination. How long will it take for the train to travel 180 miles?

$$\frac{120 \; miles}{3 \; hours} = \frac{180 \; miles}{x \; hours}$$

It is important to set up the equation so that types of quantities are in the same position in the fraction. For example, above, miles are in the numerator and hours are in the denominator. Now, solve for the missing quantity through cross-multiplication:

$$(120 \; miles) * (x \; hours) = (3 \; hours) * (180 \; miles)$$

$$x \; hours = \frac{(3 \; hours) * (180 \; miles)}{120 \; miles}$$

$x = \textbf{4.5 hours}$

One acre of wheat requires 500 gallons of water. How many acres can be watered with 2600 gallons?

This is a direct proportion – an increase in wheat requires an increase in gallons of water. Therefore it can be solved using a fraction equation:

$$\frac{1 \; acre}{500 \; gallons} = \frac{x \; acres}{2600 \; gallons}$$

$$x \; acres = \frac{(1 \; acre) * (2600 \; gallons)}{500 \; gallons}$$

$$x = \frac{26}{5} \; acres, \text{ or } \textbf{5.2 acres}$$

Check the answer – is it more or less acres than the initial value? It should be more, since there was an increase in the amount of water.

The price of a product is inversely proportional to how many are produced. If 100 products are made, they each cost $5. If 200 are made, they each cost $2.50. How much will each product cost if 400 are produced?

Inversely proportional means that as one quantity increases, the other decreases. To solve an inversely proportional problem, figure out how much one quantity goes down as the other rises.

In this example, when the number of products doubles, the price divides by 2. Therefore when quantity goes from 200 to 400, the price should go from $2.50 to $2.50/2 = **$1.25**.

Jason has realized that when more people are using his school's wifi connection, the internet speed is reduced. When there are 20 users, the speed is 3 megabits per second. When there are 60 users, the speed drops to 2 megabits per second. If the speed is inversely proportional to the number of users, what speed should Jason expect when 80 users are logged in?

To solve, first examine the rates at which the two quantities change:

When the number of users tripled from 20 to 60, the speed was reduced by $1/3^{rd}$. So if the number of users in increased by a factor of 4, how much will speed be reduced by? Solve using a fractional equation:

$$\frac{3}{1/3} = \frac{4}{x}$$

$$x = \frac{4}{3} * \frac{1}{3} = \frac{4}{9}$$

When the amount of users is multiplied by 4, the speed should reduce by 4/9. Therefore, the new speed will be:

$3 - (4/9)*3 =$ **1.67 megabits per second**.

Military Time

Many health-care facilities operate 24 hours a day, and so do not simply work "9 to 5."

To avoid time confusion – "When you say 5:00, do you mean 'am' or 'pm'?" – hospitals use military time. This might be confusing at first, but is simple once you get the hang of it.

The hours of a day start at 0000, and move through 2300. For example, 7:00 am would be 0700, because it is the 7th hour of the day. Thirty minutes later, at 7:30 am, the time would be 0730 hours.

People new to military time often get confused over the hours after noon.

Instead of 1:00 pm, military time is 1300 hours. The easiest solution to determining military time is to subject "1200" from the time.

> **Example**: 1530 hours is what time? Simply subtract 1200 from 1530, and you get 330 (which equates to **3:30 pm**).

Eventually, with real world practice, people get the hang of military time within a day or two.

Common Times:

> 0000 = 12:00 am (midnight)
>
> 0100 = 1:00 am
>
> 1200 = 12:00 (noon)
>
> 1500 = 3:00 pm
>
> 2300 = 11:00 pm

Literal Equations

Equations with more than one variable. Solve in terms of one variable first.

Example: Solve for y: $4x + 3y = 3x + 2y$.

1. Combine like terms: $3y - 2y = 4x - 3x$.

2. Solve for y. **$y = -x$**.

Algebraic Equations

When simplifying or solving algebraic equations, you need to be able to utilize all math properties: exponents, roots, negatives, order of operations, etc.

1. Addition and subtraction: Only like terms can be added or subtracted. A like term is one with the same variable or combination of variables. Constants are numbers without variables attached, and those can be grouped together as well.

Examples:

Rewrite the expression $5xy + 7y + 2yz + 11xy - 5yz$

Group together xy terms, y terms, and yz terms:

$16xy + 7y - 3yz$

Find the value of x: $5x + 4y - 16 = 4x + y + 4$

Group together like terms:

$x + 3y = 20$

Then, isolate x:

$x = 20 - 3y$

2. Multiplication: First, multiply the coefficients. Then multiply the variables:

Example: Monomial * Monomial. (Remember: a variable with no exponent has an implied exponent of 1.)
- $(3x^4y^2z)(2y^4z^5) = 6x^4y^6z^6$.

Example: Monomial * Polynomial.
- $(2y^2)(y^3 + 2xy^2z + 4z) = 2y^5 + 4xy^4z + 8y^2z$

Example: Binomial * Binomial.
- $(5x + 2)(3x + 3)$. Remember: FOIL (First, Outer, Inner, Last).

  First: $5x * 3x = 15x^2$.

  Outer: $5x * 3 = 15x$.

  Inner: $2 * 3x = 6x$.

  Last: $2 * 3 = 6$.

  Combine like terms: $15x^2 + 21x + 6$.

Example: Binomial * Polynomial.
- $(x + 3)(2x^2 - 5x - 2)$.

  First Term: $x(2x^2 - 5x - 2) = 2x^3 - 5x^2 - 2x$.

  Second term: $3(2x^2 - 5x - 2) = 6x^2 - 15x - 6$.

  Added Together: $2x^3 + x^2 - 17x - 6$.

Roman Numbers

The Roman number system uses the following identities:

Roman Numeral	Value
I	1
V	5
X	10
L	50
C	100
D	500
M	1000

These 7 numerals are combined to form numbers through addition. Numerals are always arranged from greatest to least in value. For example, the number 157 would be written as:

$$100 + 50 + 5 + 1 + 1$$

CLVII

That is the standard way to write 157, even though Roman numerals could be combined in different ways to add up to that number. In standard Roman notation, the largest possible numerals have to be used to write a number. Here's another example: the number 3,621:

$$1000 + 1000 + 1000 + 500 + 100 + 10 + 10 + 1$$

MMMDCXXI

To avoid having to add four of the same numeral in a row, subtraction is used. If a numeral with a smaller value is placed *before* a numeral with a larger value, the smaller number is subtracted from the bigger number. For example:

$$IX = 10 - 1 = 9$$

Since I has a value of 1 and it is placed *before* X, which has a value of 10, the number is found by subtracting 1 from 10. Here are a few Roman numeral example problems:

Express the number 538 in Roman Numerals.

$$538 = 500 + 30 + 8$$

$$538 = 500 + 10 + 10 + 10 + 5 + 1 + 1 + 1$$

$$538 = DXXXVIII$$

What number is expressed by the Roman Numeral CDVII?

C = 100, D = 500, V = 5, I = 1, I = 1

Since C is *before* D, 100 is subtracted from 500

500 – 100 + 5 + 1 + 1 = 407

Decimals

When adding and subtracting decimals, line up the numbers so that the decimals are aligned. You want to subtract the 1s place from the 1s place, the 1/10th place from the 1/10th place, etc. Addition follows the same rules. For example:

Find the sum of 17.07 and 2.52.

$$\begin{array}{r} 17.07 \\ +\quad 2.52 \\ =\quad \mathbf{19.59} \end{array}$$

Jeannette has 7.4 gallons of gas in her tank. After driving, she has 6.8 gallons. How many gallons of gas did she use?

$$\begin{array}{r} 7.4 \\ -\quad 6.8 \\ =\quad \mathbf{0.6\ gallons} \end{array}$$

When multiplying and dividing decimals, multiply or divide the numbers normally. Then determine the placement of the decimal point in the result by counting the number of digits after the decimal in each of the numbers you multiplied together. For example:

What is the product of 0.25 and 1.4?

25 * 14 = 350

There are 2 digits after the decimal in 0.25 and one digit after the decimal in 1.4. Therefore the product should have 3 digits after the decimal: **0.350** is the correct answer.

Determining the placement of the decimal point after division is simpler. Remember that with division, you can multiply the divisor and the dividend by any number as long as you multiply them by the same number, since those will cancel out. Change the divisor (the number you are dividing *by*) by moving the decimal point until it is a whole number. Then move the decimal point for the dividend (the number you are dividing) the same number of spaces in the same direction. After that, you can easily divide the new numbers normally to get the correct answer. For example:

Find 0.8 ÷ 0.2.

Change 0.2 to 2. The decimal moves on space to the right to accomplish this.

Next, move the decimal one space to the right on the dividend. 0.8 becomes 8.

Now, divide 8 by 2. 8/2 = **4**, which is the correct answer.

Find the quotient when 40 is divided by 0.25.

First, change the divisor to a whole number. 0.25 becomes 25.

Next, change the dividend to match the divisor. We moved the decimal two spaces to the right, so 40 becomes 4000.

4000/25 = **160**, which is correct.

Converting percentages, fractions, and decimals

This can be intimidating to some people since we are all used to simply punching in numbers into a calculator. Some are easy just because it's common knowledge for most folks that ½ equals 0.5 and ¼ equals 0.25 and so on. But how do you express a number like 3/16 in decimal form? That number probably doesn't just pop into your head for some people, but they might be able to figure it out. Others might be totally lost.

The easiest way to solve this problem is to set up a simple equation. Let's use the example 3/16.

3/16 is basically the same as saying 3 divided by 16, so let's set up that equation just like that:

$$16\overline{)3.0}$$

How many times 16 go into 3? Zero times obviously, which is why we add the decimal. Imagine the decimal isn't there, and think of it as the lowest number possible that is still bigger than 16, which is 30. So, how many times does 16 go into 30? Just 1 time, so the next step:

$$16\overline{)\begin{array}{r} 1 \\ 3.0 \\ 14.0 \end{array}}$$

Now, of course we have a remainder we have to take care of in the next step. The remainder is 14, and since 14 is smaller than 16, we need to add a decimal and think of it as 140. So, how many times does 16 go into 140? The answer is 8 times. 8 times 16 equals 128, so 140-128 means we have another remainder of 12 this time.

$$16\overline{)\begin{array}{r} 1\,8 \\ 3.0 \\ 14.0 \\ \hline 12 \end{array}}$$

Once again, think of the 12 as 120 since 16 is bigger than 12. How many times does 16 go into 120? The answer is 7 with a remainder of 8.

$$\begin{array}{r} 187 \\ 16\overline{)3.0} \\ 14.0 \\ \hline 12 \\ 8.0 \\ \hline \end{array}$$

The final step is we know that 16 can go into 80 exactly five times, so the final number = 5.

$$\begin{array}{r} 1875 \\ 16\overline{)3.0} \\ 14.0 \\ \hline 12 \\ 8.0 \\ \hline \end{array}$$

The decimal will go in front of our answer, so we now know that 3/16 = 0.1875. On the real test, you'll get a mix of hard and easy ones. One of the best ways to prepare is to simply memorize as many fractions and their decimal equivalents as you can. If you already know that 5/8 is 0.625, you don't have to spend any time on that question working it out.

Another helpful trick is to approximate. Using 5/8 as an example again, we know that 4/8 is half or 0.50 so any answer choice less than 0.5 can be eliminated. We know 6/8 is the same as ¾ or 0.75, so anything above .75 can be eliminated as well. This can many times show you the right answer without having to work it out all the way. Also, you may not need to work the problem all the way out like we did in the example to .1875 since sometimes you'll see no other answer choice even starts with the 0.18xx.

A final helpful trick is if the denominator is easily divisible by 100, you can quickly find the answer. For example, 9/20. We know 20 goes into 100 five times, so 9x5=45. Move the decimal and you have the answer of 0.45! It obviously doesn't work that easily if the denominator is 13 or 17 or another number that is not easily divisible by 100, but this method is very useful to keep in mind.

Decimals into Fraction

Many people find converting decimals into fractions easier. We have this review section after "fractions into decimals" because it is best to get the hard stuff out of the way first.

First, we need to review a basic important aspect of decimals, which are the units following the decimal. Look at this example:

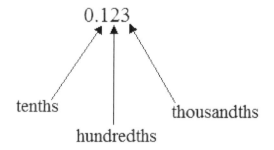

Here we see a zero with a decimal and three numbers after it. The first one is the "tenths" place, then the "hundredths", and the third one is the "thousandths". This is important to remember for solving decimal to fraction problems.

Let's work through an example: Convert 0.45 into a fraction.

Step 1: we see that this decimal number only goes to the "hundredths" place. This step almost seems to easy, but we simply start with:

$$\frac{45}{100}$$

Step 2: The next step is to simply reduce the fraction down to the lowest common denominator. For example, we know both 45 and 100 are divisible by 5, so start there. 45 divided by 5 is 9. 100 divided by 5 is 20. Therefore, we are left with:

$$\frac{9}{20}$$

And that's it! The answer is 9/20. In some cases, you might need to reduce a little further in case you accidentally did not start with the lowest common denominator. Now all that is left is to practice and you'll have the hang of it in no time. A great way to practice is to simply make your own questions since these are so straightforward unlike word problems. You can easily check yourself with an online conversion calculator if you aren't sure, and you will be a pro in no time.

Units of Measurement

You are expected to memorize some units of measurement. These are all given below:

United States Customary System	
Length	
1 foot	12 inches
1 yard	3 feet
Weight	
1 pound	16 ounces
1 ton	2000 pounds
Capacity	
1 pint	2 cups
1 quart	2 pints
1 quart	4 cups
1 gallon	4 quarts
1 gallon	8 pints
1 gallon	16 cups

Units of Time	
1 minute	60 seconds
1 hour	60 minutes
1 day	24 hours
1 week	7 days
1 year	365 days
1 year	52 weeks
1 year	12 months

Metric System	
Length	
1 kilometer	1000 meters
1 meter	100 centimeters
1 meter	1000 millimeters
1 centimeter	10 millimeters
Weight	
1 kilogram	1000 grams
1 gram	1000 milligrams
Capacity	
1 liter	1000 milliliters
1 millimeter	1 cubic centimeter

The metric system uses a standard set of prefixes that can apply to length, weight, and capacity. The most common ones are:

kilo – 1000

centi – 100

milli – 1/1000

When doing unit conversion problems, find the conversion factor. Then apply that factor to the given measurement to find the new measurement. Examples are shown below.

Practice problems:

A fence measures 15 feet long. How many yards long is the fence?

1 yard = 3 feet

15 / 3 = **5 yards**

A pitcher can hold 24 cups. How many gallons can it hold?

1 gallon = 16 cups

24 / 16 = **1.5 gallons**

A spool of wire holds 144 inches of wire. If Mario has three spools, how many feet of wire does he have?

12 inches = 1 foot

144 / 12 = 12 feet

12 feet * 3 spools = **36 feet of wire**

A ball rolling across a table travels 6 inches per second. How many feet will it travel in one minute?

This problem can be worked in two steps: finding how many inches in one minute, and then converting that to feet. It can also be worked the opposite way, by finding how many feet it travels in one second and then converting that to feet traveled per minute. The first method is shown below.

1 minute = 60 seconds

6 inches/second * 60 seconds = 360 inches

41

1 foot = 12 inches

360 inches/12 inches = **30 feet**

How many millimeters are in 0.5 meters?

1 meter = 1000 millimeters

0.5 meters = **500 millimeters**

A lead ball weighs 38 grams. How many kilograms does it weigh?

1 kilogram = 1000 grams

38 grams / 1000 grams = **0.038 kilograms**

How many cubic centimeters are in 10 liters?

1 liter = 1000 cubic centimeters

10 liters = 1000 * 10 cubic centimeters

10 liters = **10,000 cubic centimeters**

Jennifer's pencil was initially 10 centimeters long. After she sharpened it, it was 9.6 centimeters long. How many millimeters did she lose from her pencil by sharpening it?

1 centimeter = 10 millimeters

10 cm – 9.6 cm = 0.4 cm lost

0.4 centimeters = 10 * .4 millimeters = **4 millimeters** were lost

Comparison of rational numbers

Number comparison problems present numbers in different formats and ask which is larger or smaller, or whether the numbers are equivalent. The important step in solving these problems is to convert the numbers to the same format so that it is easier to see how they compare. If numbers are given in the same format, or after they have been converted, see which number is smaller or if the numbers are equal. Remember that for negative numbers, higher numbers are smaller.

Examples:

Is $4\frac{3}{4}$ greater than, equal to, or less than $\frac{18}{4}$?

These numbers are in different formats – one is a mixed fraction and the other is just a fraction. The first step is to convert the mixed fraction to a fraction:

$$4\frac{3}{4} = 4 * \frac{4}{4} + \frac{3}{4} = \frac{19}{4}$$

Once the mixed number is converted, it is easier to see that $\frac{19}{4}$ is **greater than** $\frac{18}{4}$.

Which of the following numbers has the greatest value: 104.56, 104.5, or 104.6?

These numbers are all already in the same format, so the decimal values just need to be compared. Remember that 0s can be added after the decimal without changing the value, so the three numbers can be rewritten as:

104.56

104.50

104.60

From this list, it is clearer to see that **104.60** is the greatest because .60 is larger than .50 and .56.

Is 65% greater than, less than, or equal to $\frac{13}{20}$?

The first step is to convert the numbers into the same format. 65% is the same as $\frac{65}{100}$. Next, the fractions need to be converted to have the same denominator. It is difficult to compare fractions with different denominators. Using a factor of $\frac{5}{5}$ on the second fraction will give common denominators:

$\frac{13}{20} * \frac{5}{5} = \frac{65}{100}$. Now, is easy to see that the numbers are equivalent.

Chapter 2: Reading

The Reading section measures your ability to understand, analyze, and evaluate written passages. The passages will contain material from a variety of sources, and will cover a number of different topics.

The Main Idea

Finding and understanding the main idea of a text is an essential reading skill. When you look past the facts and information and get to the heart of what the writer is trying to say, that's the **main idea**.

Imagine that you're at a friend's home for the evening:

> "Here," he says, "Let's watch this movie."

> "Sure," you reply. "What's it about?"

You'd like to know a little about what you'll be watching, but your question may not get you a satisfactory answer, because you've only asked about the subject of the film. The subject—what the movie is about—is only half the story. Think, for example, about all the alien invasion films ever been made. While these films may share the same general subject, what they have to say about the aliens or about humanity's theoretical response to invasion may be very different. Each film has different ideas it wants to convey about a subject, just as writers write because they have something they want to say about a particular subject. When you look beyond the facts and information to what the writer really wants to say about his or her subject, you're looking for the main idea.

One of the most common questions on reading comprehension exams is, "What is the main idea of this passage?" How would you answer this question for the paragraph below?

> "Wilma Rudolph, the crippled child who became an Olympic running champion, is an inspiration for us all. Born prematurely in 1940, Wilma spent her childhood battling illness, including measles, scarlet fever, chicken pox, pneumonia, and polio, a crippling disease which at that time had no cure. At the age of four, she was told she would never walk again. But Wilma and her family refused to give up. After years of special treatment and physical therapy, 12-year-old Wilma was able to walk normally again. But walking wasn't enough for Wilma, who was determined to be an athlete. Before long, her talent earned her a spot in the 1956 Olympics, where she earned a bronze medal. In the 1960 Olympics, the height of her career, she won three gold medals."

What is the main idea of this paragraph? You might be tempted to answer, "Wilma Rudolph" or "Wilma Rudolph's life." Yes, Wilma Rudolph's life is the **subject** of the passage—who or what the passage is about—but the subject is not necessarily the main idea. The **main idea** is what the writer wants to say about this subject. What is the main thing the writer says about Wilma's life?

Which of the following statements is the main idea of the paragraph?

    a) Wilma Rudolph was very sick as a child.
    b) Wilma Rudolph was an Olympic champion.
    c) Wilma Rudolph is someone to admire.

Main idea: The overall fact, feeling, or thought a writer wants to convey about his or her subject.

The best answer is **c)**: Wilma Rudolph is someone to admire. This is the idea the paragraph adds up to; it's what holds all of the information in the paragraph together. This example also shows two important characteristics of a main idea:

1. It is **general** enough to encompass all of the ideas in the passage.

2. It is an **assertion.** An assertion is a statement made by the writer.

The main idea of a passage must be general enough to encompass all of the ideas in the passage. It should be broad enough for all of the other sentences in that passage to fit underneath it, like people under an umbrella. Notice that the first two options, "Wilma Rudolph was very sick as a child" and "Wilma Rudolph was an Olympic champion", are too specific to be the main idea. They aren't broad enough to cover all of the ideas in the passage, because the passage talks about both her illnesses and her Olympic achievements. Only the third answer is general enough to be the main idea of the paragraph.

A main idea is also some kind of **assertion** about the subject. An assertion is a claim that something is true. Assertions can be facts or opinions, but in either case, an assertion should be supported by specific ideas, facts, and details. In other words, the main idea makes a general assertion that tells readers that something is true.

The supporting sentences, on the other hand, show readers that this assertion is true by providing specific facts and details. For example, in the Wilma Rudolph paragraph, the writer makes a general assertion: "Wilma Rudolph, the crippled child who became an Olympic running champion, is an inspiration for us all." The other sentences offer specific facts and details that prove why Wilma Rudolph is an inspirational person.

Writers often state their main ideas in one or two sentences so that readers can have a very clear understanding about the main point of the passage. A sentence that expresses the main idea of a paragraph is called a **topic sentence.**

Notice, for example, how the first sentence in the Wilma Rudolph paragraph states the main idea:

    "Wilma Rudolph, the crippled child who became an Olympic running champion, is an inspiration for us all."

This sentence is therefore the topic sentence for the paragraph. Topic sentences are often found at the beginning of paragraphs. Sometimes, though, writers begin with specific supporting details and lead up to the main idea, and in this case the topic sentence is often found at the end of the paragraph. Sometimes the topic sentence is even found somewhere in the middle, and other times there isn't a clear topic sentence at all—but that doesn't mean there isn't a main idea; the author has just chosen not to express it in a clear topic sentence. In this last case, you'll have to look carefully at the paragraph for clues about the main idea.

Main Ideas vs. Supporting Details

If you're not sure whether something is a main idea or a supporting detail, ask yourself the following question: Is the sentence making a **general statement**, or is it providing **specific information**? In the Wilma Rudolph paragraph above, for example, all of the sentences except the first make specific statements. They are not general enough to serve as an umbrella or net for the whole paragraph.

Writers often provide clues that can help you distinguish between main ideas and their supporting details. Here are some of the most common words and phrases used to introduce specific examples:

1. **For example…**

2. **Specifically…**

3. **In addition…**

4. **Furthermore…**

5. **For instance…**

6. **Others…**

7. **In particular…**

8. **Some…**

These signal words tell you that a supporting fact or detail will follow. If you're having trouble finding the main idea of a paragraph, try eliminating sentences that begin with these phrases because they will most likely be too specific to be a main ideas.

Implied Main Idea

When the main idea is **implied**, there's no topic sentence, which means that finding the main idea requires some detective work. But don't worry! You already know the importance of structure, word choice, style, and tone. Plus, you know how to read carefully to find clues, and you know that these clues will help you figure out the main idea.

For Example:

"One of my summer reading books was *The Windows of Time*. Though it's more than 100 pages long, I read it in one afternoon. I couldn't wait to see what happened to Evelyn, the main character. But by the time I got to the end, I wondered if I should

47

have spent my afternoon doing something else. The ending was so awful that I completely forgot that I'd enjoyed most of the book."

There's no topic sentence here, but you should still be able to find the main idea. Look carefully at what the writer says and how she says it. What is she suggesting?

    a) *The Windows of Time* is a terrific novel.
    b) *The Windows of Time* is disappointing.
    c) *The Windows of Time* is full of suspense.
    d) *The Windows of Time* is a lousy novel.

The correct answer is **b)** – the novel is disappointing. How can you tell that this is the main idea? First, we can eliminate choice **c)**, because it's too specific to be a main idea. It deals only with one specific aspect of the novel (its suspense).

Sentences **a)**, **b)**, and **d)**, on the other hand, all express a larger idea – a general assertion about the quality of the novel. But only one of these statements can actually serve as a "net" for the whole paragraph. Notice that while the first few sentences praise the novel, the last two criticize it. Clearly, this is a mixed review.

Therefore, the best answer is **b)**. Sentence **a)** is too positive and doesn't account for the "awful" ending. Sentence **d)**, on the other hand, is too negative and doesn't account for the reader's sense of suspense and interest in the main character. But sentence **b)** allows for both positive and negative aspects – when a good thing turns bad, we often feel disappointed.

Now let's look at another example. Here, the word choice will be more important, so read carefully.

> "Fortunately, none of Toby's friends had ever seen the apartment where Toby lived with his mother and sister. Sandwiched between two burnt-out buildings, his two-story apartment building was by far the ugliest one on the block. It was a real eyesore: peeling orange paint (orange!), broken windows, crooked steps, crooked everything. He could just imagine what his friends would say if they ever saw this poor excuse for a building."

Which of the following expresses the main idea of this paragraph?

    a) Toby wishes he could move to a nicer building.
    b) Toby wishes his dad still lived with them.
    c) Toby is glad none of his friends know where he lives.
    d) Toby is sad because he doesn't have any friends.

From the description, we can safely assume that Toby doesn't like his apartment building and wishes he could move to a nicer building **a)**. But that idea isn't general enough to cover the whole paragraph, because it's about his building.

Because the first sentence states that Toby has friends, the answer cannot be **d)**. We know that Toby lives only with his mother and little sister, so we might assume that he wishes his dad still lived with them, **b)**, but there's nothing in the paragraph to support that assumption, and this idea doesn't include the two main topics of the paragraph—Toby's building and Toby's friends.

What the paragraph adds up to is that Toby is terribly embarrassed about his building, and he's glad that none of his friends have seen it **c)**. This is the main idea. The paragraph opens with the word "fortunately," so we know that he thinks it's a good thing none of his friends have been to his house. Plus, notice how the building is described: "by far the ugliest on the block," which says a lot since it's stuck "between two burnt-out buildings." The writer calls it an "eyesore," and repeats "orange" with an exclamation point to emphasize how ugly the color is. Everything is "crooked" in this "poor excuse for a building." Toby is clearly ashamed of where he lives and worries about what his friends would think if they saw it.

Cause and Effect

Understanding cause and effect is important for reading success. Every event has at least one cause (what made it happen) and at least one effect (the result of what happened). Some events have more than one cause, and some have more than one effect. An event is also often part of a chain of causes and effects. Causes and effects are usually signaled by important transitional words and phrases.

Words Indicating Cause:

1. **Because (of)**

2. **Created (by)**

3. **Caused (by)**

4. **Since**

Words Indicating Effect:

1. **As a result**

2. **Since**

3. **Consequently**

4. **So**

5. **Hence**

6. **Therefore**

Sometimes, a writer will offer his or her opinion about why an event happened when the facts of the cause(s) aren't clear. Or a writer may predict what he or she thinks will happen because of a certain event (its effects). If this is the case, you need to consider how reasonable those opinions are. Are the writer's ideas logical? Does the writer offer support for the conclusions he or she offers?

Context Clues

The most fundamental vocabulary skill is using the context of a word to determine its meaning. Your ability to observe sentences closely is extremely useful when it comes to understanding new vocabulary words.

Types of Context

There are two different types of context that can help you understand the meaning of unfamiliar words: **sentence context** and **situational context**. Regardless of which context is present, these types of questions are not really testing your knowledge of vocabulary; rather, they test your ability to comprehend the meaning of a word through its usage.

Situational context is context that comes from understanding the situation in which a word or phrase occurs.

Sentence context occurs within the sentence that contains the vocabulary word. To figure out words using sentence context clues, you should first determine the most important words in the sentence.

Example: I had a hard time reading her <u>illegible</u> handwriting.
a) Neat.
b) Unsafe.
c) Sloppy.
d) Educated.

Already, you know that this sentence is discussing something that is hard to read. Look at the word that **illegible** is describing: **handwriting**. Based on context clues, you can tell that illegible means that her handwriting is hard to read.

Next, look at the answer choices. Choice **a) Neat** is obviously a wrong answer because neat handwriting would not be difficult to read. Choice **b) Unsafe** and **d) Educated** don't make sense. Therefore, choice **c) Sloppy** is the best answer choice.

Types of Clues

There are four types of clues that can help you understand context, and therefore the meaning of a word. They are **restatement**, **positive/negative**, **contrast**, and **specific detail**.

Restatement clues occur when the definition of the word is clearly stated in the sentence.

Example: The dog was <u>dauntless</u> in the face of danger, braving the fire to save the girl.
a) Difficult.
b) Fearless.
c) Imaginative.
d) Pleasant.

Demonstrating **bravery** in the face of danger would be **fearless,** choice **b)**. In this case, the context clues tell you exactly what the word means.

Positive/negative clues can tell you whether a word has a positive or negative meaning.

Example: The magazine gave a great review of the fashion show, stating the clothing was **sublime**.
a) Horrible.
b) Exotic.
c) Bland
d) Gorgeous.

The sentence tells us that the author liked the clothing enough to write a **great** review, so you know that the best answer choice is going to be a positive word. Therefore, you can immediately rule out choices **a)** and **c)** because they are negative words. **Exotic** is a neutral word; alone, it doesn't inspire a **great** review. The most positive word is gorgeous, which makes choice **d) Gorgeous** the best answer.

The following sentence uses both restatement and positive/negative clues:

"Janet suddenly found herself <u>destitute</u>, so poor she could barely afford to eat."

The second part of the sentence clearly indicates that destitute is a negative word; it also restates the meaning: very poor.

Contrast clues include the opposite meaning of a word. Words like **but, on the other hand,** and **however** are tip-offs that a sentence contains a contrast clue.

Example: Beth did not spend any time preparing for the test, but Tyron kept a <u>rigorous</u> study schedule.
a) Strict.
b) Loose.
c) Boring.
d) Strange.

In this case, the word **but** tells us that Tyron studied in a different way than Beth. If Beth did not study very hard, then Tyron did study hard for the test. The best answer here, therefore, is choice **a) Strict**.

Specific detail clues give a precise detail that can help you understand the meaning of the word.

Example: The box was heavier than he expected and it began to become <u>cumbersome</u>.

> a) Impossible.
> b) Burdensome.
> c) Obligated.
> d) Easier.

Start by looking at the specific details of the sentence. Choice **d)** can be eliminated right away because it is doubtful it would become **easier** to carry something that is **heavier**. There are also no clues in the sentence to indicate he was **obligated** to carry the box, so choice **c)** can also be disregarded. The sentence specifics, however, do tell you that the package was cumbersome because it was heavy to carry; something heavy to carry is a burden, which is **burdensome**, choice **b)**.

It is important to remember that more than one of these clues can be present in the same sentence. The more there are, the easier it will be to determine the meaning of the word, so look for them.

Denotation and Connotation

As you know, many English words have more than one meaning. For example, the word **quack** has two distinct definitions: the sound a duck makes; and a person who publicly pretends to have a skill, knowledge, education, or qualification which they do not possess.

The **denotations** of a word are the dictionary definitions.

The **connotations** of a word are the implied meaning(s) or emotion which the word makes you think.

> **Example**: "Sure," Pam said excitedly, "I'd just love to join your club; it sounds so exciting!"

Now, read this sentence:

"Sure," Pam said sarcastically, "I'd just love to join your club; it sounds so exciting!"

Even though the two sentences only differ by one word, they have completely different meanings. The difference, of course, lies in the words "excitedly" and "sarcastically."

Purpose and Tone

Whenever a person reads a text, he/she must first determine the purpose of the text. An author's purpose for writing the text can include entertainment, information, and persuasion.

Texts meant to inform should be grounded in facts and should provide empirical evidence. These texts supply data and allow the reader to form his/her own conclusions. Texts intended to persuade are when the reader is compelled to purchase something, vote for someone, or believe something.

When writing persuasive texts, authors typically employ biased language and words with distinctive connotations in order to sway the reader. This word selection and positive or negative connotation also illustrates the tone of the text. The tone is simply the writer's attitude reflected through the text.

Words that have a positive connotation usually indicate that the author approves of, respects, and/or advocates for a certain subject. Words with positive connotations include words like *brilliant* and *compassionate*. Positive connotations also typically indicate an optimistic tone.

Contrastingly, words with negative connotations usually indicate that the author disproves of, rejects, and/or dislikes a certain subject. Words with negative connotations include words like *reckless* and *excessive*. Negative connotations also typically indicate a pessimistic tone.

Fact and Opinion

As a reader, you must critically analyze the text. Ask yourself, "Is this fact or opinion?" "Are the supporting details reliable and valid?" Answering these questions will help you decide if the author is trustworthy and if the argument is coherent.

A fact is something that has been proven to be true. Gravity and tectonic plate movement are both facts; they have been proven to be true. An opinion is an assumption or something that cannot be proven to be true. Statements about personal preferences in movies and music are opinions; they cannot be proven to be true.

Identifiable factors such as weight, length, etc. are usually associated with fact. The athlete weighs 150 pounds, and the pool is 20 feet long are examples of facts determined by measureable data.

Contrastingly, words that convey degrees of being are usually associated with opinion: *good*, *better*, *best* and *bad*, *worse*, and *worst*. Red apples taste better than green apples, and this painting is the worst are both examples of opinions. Also, words that reflect abstract ideas and emotion are also associated with opinion: *love*, *friendship*, and *jealousy*.

Reading Between the Lines

Paying attention to word choice is particularly important when the main idea of a passage isn't clear. A writer's word choice doesn't just affect meaning; it also creates it. For example, look at the following description from a teacher's evaluation of a student applying to a special foreign language summer camp. There's no topic sentence, but if you use your powers of observation, you should be able to tell how the writer feels about her subject.

> "As a student, Jane usually completes her work on time and checks it carefully. She speaks French well and is learning to speak with less of an American accent. She has often been a big help to other students who are just beginning to learn the language."

What message does this passage send about Jane? Is she the best French student the writer has ever had? Is she one of the worst, or is she just average? To answer these questions, you have to make an inference, and you must support your inference with specific observations. What makes you come to the conclusion that you come to?

The **diction** of the paragraph above reveals that this is a positive evaluation, but not a glowing recommendation.

Here are some of the specific observations you might have made to support this conclusion:

- The writer uses the word "usually" in the first sentence. This means that Jane is good about meeting deadlines for work, but not great; she doesn't always hand in her work on time.

- The first sentence also says that Jane checks her work carefully. While Jane may sometimes hand in work late, at least she always makes sure it's quality work. She's not sloppy.

- The second sentence tells us she's "learning to speak with less of an American accent." This suggests that she has a strong accent and needs to improve in this area. It also suggests, though, that she is already making progress.

- The third sentence tells us that she "often" helps "students who are just beginning to learn the language." From this we can conclude that Jane has indeed mastered the basics. Otherwise, how could she be a big help to students who are just starting to learn? By looking at the passage carefully, then, you can see how the writer feels about her subject.

Summarizing

Often, students make summarizing more complicated than it needs to be. Selecting the correct summary is quite simple. Simply ensure that the summary:

1. States the main ideas from the beginning, middle, and end of the text.
2. Follows the sequence of events as reflected in the text.
3. Uses accurate information from the text.

When answering questions related to summarizing, remember to read the text carefully, and then eliminate the incorrect answer choices by checking for the criteria listed above.

Key Terms

Antonym - a word that has an opposite meaning of another word
Assumption - an idea or statement thought to be true
Connotation - an implied meaning of a word
Context clue - clues within the text that provide hints of the meaning of a word or phrase
Inference - a logical judgment made after reading a phrase or sentence in a text
Synonym - a word that has a similar meaning to another word
Tone - the character of the text in terms of word choice, sentence structure, etc.

Test Your Knowledge: Reading Review Quiz

Read each of the following paragraphs carefully and answer the questions that follow.

My "office" measures a whopping 5 x 7 feet. A large desk is squeezed into one corner, leaving just enough room for a rickety chair between the desk and the wall. Yellow paint is peeling off the walls in dirty chunks. The ceiling is barely six feet tall; it's like a hat that I wear all day long. The window, a single 2 x 2 pane, looks out onto a solid brick wall just two feet away.

1. What is the main idea implied by this paragraph?
    a) This office is small but comfortable.
    b) This office is in need of repair.
    c) This office is old and claustrophobic.
    d) None of the above.

There are many things you can do to make tax time easier. The single most important strategy is to keep accurate records. Keep all of your pay stubs, receipts, bank statements, and other relevant financial information in a neat, organized folder so that when you're ready to prepare your form, all of your paperwork is in one place. The second thing you can do is start early. Get your tax forms from the post office as soon as they are available and start calculating. This way, if you run into any problems, you have plenty of time to straighten them out. You can also save time by reading the directions carefully. This will prevent time-consuming errors. Finally, if your taxes are relatively simple (you don't have itemized deductions or special investments), use the shorter tax form. It's only one page, so if your records are in order, it can be completed in less than an hour.

2. The sentence "It's only one page, so if your records are in order, it can be completed in less than an hour" is:
    a) The main idea of the passage.
    b) A major supporting detail.
    c) A minor supporting detail.
    d) A transitional sentence.

3. A good summary of this passage would be:
    a) Simple strategies can make tax time less taxing.
    b) Don't procrastinate at tax time.
    c) Always keep good records.
    d) Get a tax attorney.

Being a secretary is a lot like being a parent. After a while, your boss becomes dependent upon you, just as a child is dependent upon his or her parents. Like a child who must ask permission before going out, you'll find your boss coming to you for permission, too. "Can I have a meeting on Tuesday at 3:30?" you might be asked, because you're the one who keeps track of your boss's schedule. You will also find yourself cleaning up after your boss a lot, tidying up papers and files the same way a parent tucks away a child's toys and clothes. And, like a parent protects his or her children from outside dangers, you will find yourself protecting your boss from certain "dangers"— unwanted callers, angry clients, and upset subordinates.

4. The main idea of this passage is:
   a) Secretaries are treated like children.
   b) Bosses treat their secretaries like children.
   c) Secretaries and parents have similar roles.
   d) Bosses depend too much upon their secretaries.

5. Which of the following is the topic sentence of the paragraph?
   a) Being a secretary is a lot like being a parent.
   b) After a while, your boss becomes dependent upon you, just as a child is dependent upon his or her parents.
   c) You will also find yourself cleaning up after your boss a lot, tidying up papers and files the same way a parent tucks away a child's toys and clothes.
   d) None of the above.

6. The tone of this passage suggests that:
   a) The writer is angry about how secretaries are treated.
   b) The writer thinks secretaries do too much work.
   c) The writer is slightly amused by how similar the roles of secretaries and parents are.
   d) The writer is both a secretary and a parent.

7. The sentence, "'Can't I have a meeting on Tuesday at 3:30?' you might be asked, because you're the one who keeps track of your boss's schedule," is a:
   a) Main idea.
   b) Major supporting detail.
   c) Minor supporting detail.
   d) None of the above.

Use context clues to determine the meaning of each underlined word.

8. His story didn't seem very realistic; even though it was a documentary.
   a) Believable.
   b) Humorous.
   c) Poetic.
   d) Exciting.

9. Listening to music too loudly, especially through headphones, can impair your hearing.
   a) Damage.
   b) Heighten.
   c) Use.
   d) Ensure.

10. Kelly's game happened to coincide with the Sue's recital.
   a) Happen before.
   b) Occur at the same time.
   c) Occur afterward.
   d) Not happen.

Fill in the blank to complete the sentence.

11. Texts intended to _____ are when the reader is compelled to purchase something, vote for someone, or believe something.
    a) Inform
    b) Persuade
    c) Entertain
    d) None of the above

12. Statements about personal preferences in movies and music are _____.
    a) Facts
    b) Opinions
    c) Truths
    d) None of the above

13. A(n) _____ is a logical judgment made after reading a phrase or sentence in a text.
    a) Assumption
    b) Antonym
    c) Synonym
    d) Inference

Test Your Knowledge: Reading—Answers

1. c)

2. c)

3. a)

4. c)

5. a)
6. c)

7. c)

8. a) Believable.
   Realistic means accurate, truthful, and believable.

9. a) Damage.
   This is the only logical choice.

10. b) Occur at the same time.
    According to information in the sentence, the game was scheduled at the same time as the recital.

11. b)

12. b)

13. d)

Chapter 3: Grammar

It's time to review those basic techniques used to determine the meanings of words with which you are not familiar. Don't worry though! The good news is that you have been using various degrees of these techniques since you first began to speak.

We have not included a vocabulary list in this book, because reading definitions from a page is the worst way to improve word knowledge. Interaction, and seeing the words used in context, is the best way to learn. We recommend using flashcards to improve your vocabulary knowledge – there are many resources available online. The best we've found is www.vocabulary.com/il; but you should find what suits you specifically!

Below are techniques for improving and utilizing the vocabulary you already have.

Punctuation

You've already learned a lot about punctuation in the past, but we need to go over it again so that you do your best on your exam. Formally, the term "punctuation" refers to the use of conventional marks in writing to separate elements and make meaning clear. But you probably know about it as all those periods, commas, semicolons, hyphens, and quotation marks that fill your papers and books. Yes, the list of punctuation marks is seemingly endless – and we can't possibly review them all here – so let's touch on the basics, which will be more than enough to prepare you for the HESI A2.

Here's the opening paragraph of a very famous book, Charles Dickens' *A Tale of Two Cities*:

> It was the best of times, it was the worst of times, it was the age of wisdom, it was the age of foolishness, it was the epoch of belief, it was the epoch of incredulity, it was the season of Light, it was the season of Darkness, it was the spring of hope, it was the winter of Despair, we had everything before us, we were all going direct to Heaven, we were all going direct the other way – in short, the period was so far like the present period, that some of its noisiest authorities insisted on its being received, for good or for evil, in the superlative degree of comparison only. (1)

Dickens' paragraph contains two immediately noticeable features, which are very apparent. First, the paragraph is one-sentence long. Second, it uses three punctuation marks: the comma, the dash, and the period. As you most likely noticed, the most prevalent punctuation mark is the comma, which makes the paragraph readable and, hopefully, exciting.

But you don't find out what the "it" – a time period that is simultaneously the past and the present – is until after the dash. Dickens creates anticipation and drama by using commas to separate the adjectival clauses that describe many things: both the past and the present, as well as the book that you're about to read.

Dickens, moreover, uses commas to give his opening paragraph a sense of rhythm by directing you where to stop. Reading this paragraph out loud is a lot of fun, because you can feel the passage's rhythm as you go.

Now, let's contrast the opening paragraph of *A Tale of Two Cities* to the opening paragraph of Salman Rushdie's *Midnight's Children*, a contemporary novel. Here's Rushdie's paragraph:

I was born in the city of Bombay . . . once upon a time. No, that won't do, there's no getting away from the date: I was born in Doctor Narlikar's Nursing Home on August 15th, 1947. And the time? The time matters, too. Well then: at night. No, it's important to be more . . . On the stroke of midnight, as a matter of fact. Clock-hands joined palms in respectful greeting as I came. Oh, spell it out, spell it out: at the precise instant of India's arrival at independence, I tumbled forth into the world. There were gasps. And, outside the window, fireworks and crowds. A few seconds later, my father broke his big toe; but his accident was a mere trifle when set beside what had befallen me in that benighted moment, because thanks to the occult tyrannies of those blandly saluting clocks I had been mysteriously handcuffed to history, my destinies indissolubly chained to those of my country. For the next three decades, there was to be no escape. Soothsayers had prophesied me, newspapers celebrated my arrival, politicos ratified my authenticity. I was left entirely without a say in the matter. I, Saleem Sinai, later variously called Snotnose, Stainface, Baldy, Sniffer, Buddha and even Piece-of-the-Moon, had become heavily embroiled in Fate – at the best of times a dangerous sort of involvement. And I couldn't even wipe my own nose at the time.

You already know what's going on here. Rushdie, in comparison to Dickens, uses many punctuation marks. His paragraph includes ellipses, commas, apostrophes, colons, question marks, semicolons, and dashes. Why does he feature so many punctuation marks, and how do they impact the meaning of his paragraph?

To answer this question, we need to examine the first five sentences of the paragraph.

1. In the first sentence, Rushdie employs ellipses. This punctuation mark suggests that Saleem hesitates at the beginning of his story. After starting with a very confident statement about his birth ("I was born in the city of Bombay"), he pauses and then relies on one of the most clichéd ways to begin a story ("once upon a time"). Rushdie's use of punctuation, accordingly, tells us a lot about his narrator's timid personality.

2. The second sentence uses commas to continue to illustrate Saleem's nervousness to begin his story. The commas after "[n]o" and "oh" indicate that Saleem pauses and has a hard time getting the words out. The colon, however, suggests a full stop and prepares the reader for Saleem's second definitive statement: "I was born in Doctor Narlikar's Nursing Home on August 15th, 1947."

3. The third sentence is a question and contains the appropriate punctuation mark. Saleem anticipates a question that the reader might have and puts himself in the position of the reader. He proceeds to answer his own question in the fourth sentence, with another factual declaration about the importance of time.

4. The fifth sentence continues Saleem's seeming unwillingness to get to the point. Rushdie again uses a colon, so readers expect a definitive answer, like they got in the second sentence. But instead they get more vague information: "Well then: at night."

Do you get the point? It's that Dickens' simple but effective use of punctuation creates a solid rhythm that lends the narrative voice authority. In contrast, Rushdie's more complicated punctuation creates a tentative and even awkward narrative voice. Neither Dickens nor Rushdie is a *better* writer (you might like one paragraph more than the other – and that's okay), but they both use punctuation in amazing ways to provide crucial information about their narrators – information that impacts the way you respond to their writing.

Parts of Speech

Nouns: Nouns are people, places, or things. They are typically the subject of a sentence.

Example: "The hospital was very clean."

The noun is "hospital;" it is the "place."

Pronouns: Pronouns essentially "replace" nouns. This allows a sentence to not sound repetitive.

Example: "Sam stayed home from school because Sam was not feeling well."

The word "Sam" appears twice in the same sentence. Instead, you can use a pronoun and say, "Sam stayed at home because *he* did not feel well."

Some common pronouns include:

- I, me, mine, my
- You, your, yours
- He, him, his
- She, her, hers
- It, its
- We, us, our, ours
- They, them, their, theirs

Verbs: Verbs are the "action" of a sentence; verbs "do" things.

They can, however, be quite tricky. A verb can have many variations, depending on the subject of a sentence, the tense of the word (past, present, future, etc.), and whether or not it is regular or irregular.

Example: "He runs to second base." The verb is "runs," a regular verb.

Example: "I am 7 years old." The verb in this case is "am," an irregular verb.

As mentioned above, verbs must use the correct tense – and that tense must remain the same throughout the sentence. "I was baking cookies and eat some dough." Here, the two verbs "baking" and "eat" are presented in different tenses. "Was baking" occurred in the past; "eat" occurs in the present. Instead, it should be "ate some dough."

Adjectives: Adjectives are words that describe a noun and give more information.

Example: "The boy hit the ball."

If you want to know more about the noun "boy," you could use an adjective to describe it. "The little boy hit the ball." An adjective simply provides more information about a noun or subject in a sentence.

Adverbs: Adverbs are similar to adjectives in that they provide more information; however, they describe verbs, adjectives, and even other adverbs. They do not describe nouns, however.

Example: "The doctor said she hired a new employee."

It would give more information to say: "The doctor said she recently hired a new employee." Now we know more about *how* the action was executed. Adverbs typically describe when or how something has happened, how it looks, how it feels, etc.

Prepositions: Prepositions express the location of a noun or pronoun in relation to other words and phrases in a sentence.

Example: "The nurse parked her car in a parking garage."

The preposition "in" is describing the location of the nurse's car. A prepositional phrase is a phrase that starts with a preposition and ends with a noun. The prepositional phrase is "in a parking garage." Here, "in" is the preposition and "garage is the noun."

Conjunctions: Conjunctions connect words, phrases, and clauses. Some common conjunctions include *and, but*, and *or*.

Example: "The nurse prepared the patient for surgery, and the doctor performed the surgery."

Here, the two independent clauses "The nurse prepared the patient for surgery" and "The doctor performed the surgery" are joined by the conjunction "and."

Interjections: Interjections express emotion.

Example: "Gee, that race was close!"

"Gee" is the interjection. It shows how excited this particular person is about the race.

Important Terms

Clause - a group of words that has a subject committing an action and a predicate
Direct object - a noun or pronoun that receives the action of the verb
Indirect object - a noun or pronoun for which the action is completed
Phrase - a group of words that does not have a subject committing an action
Predicate - one of the two parts of a clause; provides information about the subject
Predicate adjective - an adjective that follows a linking verb that modifies the subject
Predicate nominative - a noun that follows a linking verb that indicates what the subject is

<u>Sentence</u> - a group of words that includes a subject and a predicate that conveys a complete thought

<u>Subject</u> - one of the two parts of a clause; is the main entity of the clause (person, place, idea, etc.)

Common Errors

Subject-Verb Agreement: The subject must agree with the verb in number. A singular noun requires a singular verb, and a plural noun requires a plural verb. Often, this is quite easy to accomplish because the subject and verb are usually quite close to each other.

"The cat (singular noun) chases (singular verb) the ball."

"The cats (plural noun) play (plural verb) at the same time."

Sometimes, the subject and verb are separated by clauses or phrases. In these instances, ignore the clauses and phrases and make sure the subject and verb agree in number.

"The cars (plural noun) that had been recalled by the manufacturer were returned (plural verb) within a few months."

Sometimes, the subject of a sentence is a collective noun. A collective noun is singular, but reflects a group of people or items. This group can reflect a single entity or separate entities. When the group reflects a single unit, use a singular verb; when the group reflects separate items, use a plural verb.

"The deer hid in the trees."

"The deer are not all the same size."

Sometimes, the subject of a sentence is a compound subject. When the subject contains two or more words connected by *and*, the subject is plural and requires a plural verb. When the subject contains two or more singular words connected by *or, either/or, neither/nor*, or *not only/but also*, the subject is singular and requires a singular verb. When the subject contains singular and plural words connected by *or, either/or, neither/nor*, or *not only/but also*, select a verb that agrees with the subject closest to it.

"The doctor and nurse (plural noun) work (plural verb) in the hospital."

"Neither the employer (singular noun) nor the employee (singular noun) was (singular verb) scheduled to take a vacation."

"Either the parents (plural noun) or the son (singular noun) was responsible (singular verb) for the success."

Comma in a Compound Sentence: A compound sentence contains two or more independent clauses. Every independent clause has a subject and a predicate and can stand alone as a sentence. When two independent clauses are connected by a coordinating conjunction, insert a comma before the conjunction.

"The dog was large, and the cat was small."

Run-On Sentence: A run-on sentence consists of two complete sentences (or independent clauses) written as only one sentence. To correct a run-on sentence, insert a semicolon between the independent clauses, add a comma and coordinating conjunction, or separate the two independent clauses into two sentences.

"The dog was large the cat was small."
→ "The dog was large; the cat was small."
→ "The dog was large, and the cat was small."
→ "The dog was large." "The cat was small."

A comma splice is an example of a run-on sentence. It is has two independent clauses connected by only a comma. To correct a comma splice, replace the comma with a semicolon, colon, or dash (depending on the sentence); add a coordinating conjunction; or separate the single sentence into two sentences.

"The nurse prepared the patient for surgery, the doctor performed the surgery."
→ "The nurse prepared the patient for surgery; the doctor performed the surgery."
→ "The nurse prepared the patient for surgery, and the doctor performed the surgery."
→ "The nurse prepared the patient for surgery." "The doctor performed the surgery."

Pronoun Case: Pronoun case is the form of a noun or pronoun that reflects its relation to other words in a sentence. The three pronoun cases are subjective, objective, and possessive. Subjective case is used when pronouns are the subject. Objective case is used when pronouns are the objects of verbs or prepositions. Possessive case is used when pronouns express ownership.

Pronouns as Subjects	Pronouns as Objects	Pronouns as Possessives
I	Me	My (Mine)
You	You	Your (Yours)
He, She, It	Him, Her, It	His, Her (Hers), It (Its)
We	Us	Our (Ours)
They	Them	Their (Theirs)
Who	Whom	Whose

There are some situations where you may be confused about which pronoun case to use. These situations include compound structures and comparisons.

Compound structures are when there is a noun and pronoun or two pronouns in a sentence. To determine the correct pronoun case in these situations, drop the noun from the sentence and check which pronoun case makes sense.

"Jackie and me play cards once a week." (*Me play cards once a week.*)
"She gave the book to Ben and I." (*She gave the book to I.*)
"Us listeners like that song." (*Us like that song.*)
If the included pronoun case makes sense, leave the sentence as is. If the included pronoun case doesn't make sense, correct the sentence. None of the sentences above make sense using the included pronoun case. So, select the correct pronoun case so the sentences make sense.

"Jackie and *I* play cards once a week." (*I play cards once a week.*)
"She gave the book to Ben and *me*." (*She gave the book to me.*)
"*We* listeners like that song." (*We like that song.*)

Comparisons are sentences that typically omit parts of sentences and follow *than* or *as*. To determine the correct pronoun case in these situations, complete the comparison and check which pronoun case makes sense.

"He is older than me." *(am)*
"She is as smart as me." *(am)*

If the included pronoun case makes sense, leave the sentence as is. If the included pronoun case doesn't make sense, correct the sentence. Neither of the sentences above makes sense using the included pronoun case. So, select the correct pronoun case so the sentences make sense.

"He is older than *I*." *(am)*
"She is as smart as *I*." *(am)*

Pronouns that Indicate Possession: Personal pronouns have specific possessive forms.

Pronoun	Possessive Pronouns
I	My, Mine
He	His, His
She	Her, Hers
We	Our, Ours
You	Your, Yours
They	Their, Theirs
It	Its, Its

Remember not to confuse possessive pronouns with contractions that are pronounced or spelled similarly.

Possessive Pronoun	Contraction
Its (belonging to *it*)	It's (it is, it has)
Their (belonging to *them*)	They're (they are)
Whose (belonging to *whom*)	Who's (who is, who has)
Your (belonging to *you*)	You're (you are)

Comma in a Series: In English, you can either use or not use a comma after the second-to-last item in a series.

"The nurse had to wash her hands, feed the client, and document the task."
"The nurse had to wash her hands, feed the client and document the task."

Technically, both sentences above are correct. However, in some cases, omitting the comma before the coordinating conjunction can confuse the reader.

"Jan enjoys the company of her parents, Suzie and Derek."

In the sentence above, are Jan's parents named Suzie and Derek? Does Jan enjoy the company of her parents and also enjoy the company of Suzie and Derek? With the comma omitted, it's hard to tell what the writer is saying.

"Jan enjoys the company of her parents, Suzie, and Derek."

In this sentence, it is quite clear that Jan enjoys the company of her parents as well as the company of Suzie and Derek. To make your writing as clear as possible, insert a comma before the coordinating conjunction when listing items in a series.

Unclear or Vague Pronoun Reference: Sometimes a pronoun may seem to reference more than one noun, which makes the sentence awkward and difficult to understand.

"The father and the son knew he had played a great game."

There are several possible interpretations of the sentence above. Did the father know his son had played a great game? Did the son know he himself had played a great game? Did the father know he himself had played a great game? Did the son know his father had played a great game? This sentence is confusing and should be rewritten.

"The father knew his son had played a great game."

In the sentence above, there is no question about the meaning. It clearly states that the father knows his son had played a great game.

Sentence Fragments: A sentence fragment is simply an incomplete sentence. Many times, a sentence fragment is a dependent clause. Dependent clauses often start with words such as *while*, *because*, *although*, *however*, and *among*. To correct sentence fragments, or dependent clauses, add an independent clause to the sentence.

"Although the nurse was on a break."
→ "Although the nurse was on a break, she returned to complete the task."

Misplaced Modifier: A misplaced modifier is a word or phrase that is inappropriately separated from the word it actually modifies. Many times, the position of the modifier makes it seem as though it modifies a word or phrase it isn't intended to modify.

"David only rode the bus for 10 minutes."
"David rode the bus for only 10 minutes."

In the first sentence, David only rode the bus; he didn't see it, he didn't hear it, and he didn't run alongside it. In the second sentence, David rode the bus for only 10 minutes; not 5 minutes, not 20 minutes, and not 30 minutes.

"Mary saw a patient in the elevator."
"Mary saw a patient while in the elevator."

In the first sentence, Mary saw a patient in the elevator; the nurse saw a patient alone enter the elevator. In the second sentence, Mary saw a patient in the elevator while she herself was in the elevator; they were both in the elevator together.

"Jennifer heard a dog in her bedroom."
"In her bedroom, Jennifer heard a dog."

In the first sentence, Jennifer heard a dog in her bedroom; the dog was in her bedroom. In the second sentence, Jennifer heard a dog from her bedroom; the dog was not necessarily in Jennifer's bedroom.

An example of a misplaced modifier is a dangling participial phrase. A participial phrase is a group of words that includes a present participle (word + *ing*) or past participle (word + *en*) and any modifiers, objects, and complements. A participial phrase usually functions as an adjective. When a participial phrase is placed either directly before or after a noun it doesn't modify, it is called a dangling participial phrase.

"Remembering the patient's feedback, the procedure was modified accordingly by the nurse."

Remembering the patient's feedback is intended to modify the noun *nurse*. However, because that phrase is placed next to *the procedure*, it seems as if *remembering the patient's feedback* is modifying *the procedure*. This suggests that *the procedure* is *remembering the patient's feedback*, which of course, is not possible.

"Remembering the patient's feedback, the nurse modified accordingly the procedure."

In the sentence above, *remembering the patient's feedback* is now placed directly before and now correctly modifies *the nurse*.

Prepositions at the End of a Sentence: Generally, it is incorrect to end a sentence with a preposition. However, correcting a sentence with a preposition at the end sometimes makes the sentence sound odd. If this occurs, it is best to rewrite the sentence to avoid the preposition at the end as well as to avoid any awkwardness.

"What are you talking about?"
"About what are you talking?"
"What are you saying?"

The first sentence above ends in a preposition. However, the second sentence sounds odd after the ending preposition is removed. The third sentence (a rewrite of the first and second sentences) makes the most sense and is grammatically correct. It does not end with a preposition, and it does not sound awkward.

Helpful Recommendations

Eliminate clichés: Clichés are words or phrases that are so overused that they have lost their original meaning. Examples include "out of this world," "second to none," and "around the clock."

Clichés may be used often when speaking English, but they are considered inappropriate when writing English. Additionally, using more descriptive phrases will strengthen your writing.

Eliminate euphemisms: A euphemism is a word of phrase used in place of another word or phrase that may be offensive or unpleasant. These include "on the street" and "passed away." Euphemisms, like clichés, are used often, but try to reduce or eliminate using them in your own writing and speaking. Using accurate language is crucial, especially in the healthcare profession.

Eliminate sexist language: Sexist language is words that carelessly highlight one gender over the other. Consider the following sentence: "A writer can write anything he chooses." This would be considered sexist language. Instead of using "he" to reflect what could be either a male or female writer, use "he or she (he/she)."

Then the sentence would read "A writer can write anything he/she chooses."

Another option in this case would be to change the singular noun "writer" to the plural noun "writers" and then change "he" to "they."

Then the sentence would read "Writers can write anything they choose."

Eliminate profanity and insensitive language: Profanity is considered to be language that is profane, vulgar, and/or threatening. Insensitive language is considered to be language that isolates a person or group of people according to race, ethnicity, age, religion, or disability. In the healthcare profession, it is especially critical to treat everyone respectfully and equally. To do otherwise would be unprofessional.

Word Pairs

The following word pairs sound alike, but are spelled and used differently. Be sure to understand the spelling and usage differences of these words.

Affect versus Effect: Generally, *affect* is used as a verb, and *effect* is used as a noun.

"This medication adversely affects the patient."
"The side effect of this medication could cause adverse reactions."

In the first sentence, *affects* is used as a verb. In the second sentence, *effect* is used as a noun.

Among versus Between: Although it is commonly believed that *between* is used for choices involving two items and *among* is used for choices involving three or more items, it is not necessarily the rule. There are three categories of rules for these two words.

Relationships:
B*etween* refers to distinctive, concrete items either in relationships with only two items or in relationships with more than two items. *Among* refers to non-individual, collective items.

"Let's keep this secret between you and me."

"There are differences between hockey, basketball, and football."
"Gossip spread among the students."

The first sentence involves two individual people (*you* and *me*), so *between* is used. The second sentence, although it involves three items (*hockey*, *basketball*, and *football*), refers to individual sports, so *between* is used. The third sentence involves a collective group (*students*), so *among* is used.

Part of a Group:
Among can indicate exclusion from a group.

"Kelly felt like a stranger among friends."
"Peter was happy to find a friend among enemies."

The first sentence reflects that Kelly feels as though she is not among the group of friends. The second sentence reflects that Peter was able to find someone not among the group of enemies.

Location:
Between and *among* can reflect different meanings when used in a sentence.

"Mike ran between the parked cars."
"Mike ran among the parked cars."

The first sentence suggests that Mike ran *between* two parked cars. The second sentence suggests that Mike ran *among* several cars, such as in a parking lot.

Amount versus Number: *Amount* is used to indicate a quantity that cannot be counted. *Number* is used to indicate a quantity that can be counted.

"The patient has lost a large amount of blood."
"The patient has undergone a number of blood transfusions."

Blood itself cannot be counted (unless it is placed in a measureable container). The number of blood transfusion procedures, however, can be counted.

Good versus Well: *Good* is an adjective and should be used as such. *Well* is an adverb and should be used as such.

"The sizzling steak was delicious."
"The student performed well."

Adjectives modify nouns. In the first sentence, *sizzling* modifies *steak*, a noun. Adverbs modify verbs. In the second sentence, *well* modifies *performed*, a verb.

Bad versus Badly: *Bad* is an adjective and should be used as such. *Badly* is an adverb and should be used as such. A helpful way to remember adjectives from adverbs is that adverbs almost always end in *ly*.

"The bad food gave me a stomach ache."
"I lost the race badly."

Adjectives modify nouns. In the first sentence, *bad* modifies the noun *food*. Adverbs modify verbs. In the second sentence, *badly* modifies the verb *lost*.

Bring versus Take: *Bring* reflects activity toward the speaker (there to here). *Take* reflects activity away from the speaker (here to there).

"Bring the car from the school to my house."
"Take the car from my house to the shop."

In the first sentence, the speaker is wants the car to be *brought* from the school to his/her location (the house). In the second sentence, the speaker wants the car to be *taken* from his/her location (the house) to the shop.

Can versus May (Could versus Might): *Can* and *could* reflect the possibility of something. *May* and *might* reflect permission to do something.

"David can enroll in college."
"Mary may have some ice cream."

In the first sentence, David has the possibility of enrolling in college; it doesn't necessarily mean he will. In the second sentence, Mary has been granted permission to eat some ice cream.

Farther versus Further: *Farther* is used to indicate a physical distance. *Further* is used to indicate a figurative distance.

"I do not wish to walk any farther."
"I do not wish to discuss this topic further."

In the first sentence, *more walking* is a physical distance, so *farther* is used. In the second sentence, *more discussion* is a figurative distance, so *further* is used.

Fewer versus Less: *Fewer* is used to indicate a countable quantity. *Less* is used to indicate an uncountable quantity.

"There are fewer apples than oranges in this basket."
"There is less water in this glass than in that bucket."

In the first sentence, you can physically count the apples and oranges. In the second sentence, there is no physical way to separate or count the water; it's simply a single volume of liquid.

Hear versus Here: *Hear* refers to the auditory sense. *Here* refers to a location.

"Jake hears the airplane overhead."
"Sarah is here at the airport with Jake."

In the first sentence, Jake listens and *hears* the airplane overhead. In the second sentence, Sarah is at the same location as Jake.

i.e. versus e.g.: *i.e.* is an abbreviation used to reinforce what is being discussed. *e.g.* is an abbreviation used to give an example of what is being discussed. A rough translation of i.e. is *in other words*. A rough translation of e.g. is *for example*.

"The car broke down, i.e. the driver had to call a taxi."
"The test was long, e.g. there were 50 questions about Calculus alone."

In the first sentence, the car broke down; *in other words*, so the driver had to call a taxi. In the second sentence, the test was long; *for example*, there were 50 Calculus questions, not to mention all the questions about other subjects.

Learn versus Teach: *Learn* means to receive or obtain knowledge and information. *Teach* means to disseminate or distribute knowledge.

"Sarah learned all about the U.S. Constitution in her history course."
"She will teach this knowledge to students in the future."

In the first sentence, Sarah *obtained* knowledge about the Constitution in her history class. In the second sentence, she will *distribute* that knowledge to students in the future.

Lay versus Lie: This word pair is extremely tricky because the past and present tenses are somewhat counterintuitive. However, regardless of the tense, the rule is that *lay* requires a direct object, whereas *lie* does not. Here are some examples of the present tense of lay and lie.

"You lay the pencil on the desk."
"You lie on the bed."

In the first sentence, pencil is the direct object, so *lay* is used. In the second sentence, there is no direct object, so *lie* is used. Another way to remember the difference between these two words is this general rule: You *lay* something down, and people *lie* down by themselves.

The past tense of lay is *laid*. The past tense of lie is *lay*.

"Last week, Susan laid the quilt on the sofa."
"Yesterday, Jim lay on the grass."

In the first sentence, quilt is the direct object, so *laid* is used. Remember, laid is the past tense of lay. In the second sentence, there is no direct object, so *lay* is used. Remember, lay is the past tense of lie. Using the general rule, Susan *laid* something down, and Jim *lay* down himself.

The past participle of lie is *lain*. The past participle of lay is *laid*.

"Margie has laid dinner on the table."
"Steve has lain in bed for a week."

In the first sentence, dinner is the direct object, so *laid* is once again used. Remember, laid is the past participle of lay. In the second sentence, there is no direct object, so *lain* is used. Remember, lain is the past participle of lie. Using the general rule, Margie has *laid* something down, and Steve has *lain* down himself.

An excellent source to refer back to in the future can be found at: http://www.quickanddirtytips.com/education/grammar/lay-versus-lie.

Which versus That: *Which* is used to start a non-essential clause. *That* is used to start an essential clause. Non-essential clauses can be removed from the sentence, and the sentence will still make sense. Essential clauses are required to understand the meaning of the sentence.

"The large house, which was on the corner, is yellow."
"The dog that has brown spots was barking."

In the first sentence, the large house is yellow. The fact that it's on the corner has nothing to do with its color. As explained above, the non-essential clause (*which was on the corner*) can be removed, and the sentence will still make sense. In the second sentence, the dog with brown spots was barking; not just any dog, but specifically, the dog with brown spots.

Who versus Whom: *Who* is used when referring to the subject of a clause. *Whom* is used when referring to the object of a clause. These words can also be thought of as the person doing or receiving an action.

"He is the person who waved at me this morning."
"She is the person whom I spoke to yesterday."

In the first sentence, *He* is the person doing an action. He waved at me. Therefore, *who* is used. In the second sentence, *She* is the person receiving an action. She was spoken to by another person. Therefore, *whom* is used.

Key Terms

Adjective - a word used to modify a noun
Adverb - a word used to modify a verb
Independent clause - a clause that expresses a complete thought and can stand as its own sentence
Dependent clause - a clause that is an incomplete thought and cannot stand as its own sentence
Cliché - an overused word or phrase that has lost its original meaning
Compound sentence - a sentence that contains at least two independent clauses
Conjunction - a word that connects two parts of a sentence
Direct object - a noun or pronoun that receives the action of the verb
Euphemism - a word of phrase used in place of another word or phrase that may be offensive or unpleasant
Indirect object - a noun or pronoun for which the action is completed
Interjection - a word that expresses emotion
Misplaced modifier - a word or phrase that is inappropriately separated from the word it modifies; many times, it modifies a word it wasn't intended to modify
Common noun - a noun that is not used as a name for a specific person, event, or place

Proper noun - a noun that is used as a name for a specific person, event, or place
Abstract noun - a noun that refers to something that a person cannot interact with physically
Collective noun - a singular noun that reflects a group of people or items
Participial phrase - a phrase that includes a participle and modifies the subject
Participle - a form of a verb that varies depending on the sentence in which it's used
Phrase - a group of words that does not have a subject committing an action
Predicate - one of the two parts of a clause; provides information about the subject
Predicate adjective - an adjective that follows a linking verb that modifies the subject
Predicate nominative - a noun that follows a linking verb that indicates what the subject is
Preposition - a word that indicates the position or location of a word or phrase
Personal pronoun - a pronoun that represents a specific person, place, group, or thing
Possessive pronoun - a pronoun that refers to a person or thing that belongs to another person; possessive pronouns must agree in number (singular or plural), person (first, second, or third), and gender (male or female)
Run-on sentence - a sentence that consists of two complete sentences (or independent clauses) written as only one sentence
Declarative sentence - a sentence that reflects a statement
Interrogative sentence - a sentence that reflects a question
Imperative sentence - a sentence that reflects a command or request
Exclamatory sentence - a sentence that reflects strong feelings or exclamation
Sentence fragment - a group of words that is used as a sentence, but is not grammatically complete; an example is a dependent clause by itself
Sexist language - words that carelessly highlight one gender over the other
Subject - one of the two parts of a clause; is main entity of the clause (person, place, idea, etc.)
Verb - a word used to reflect action

Study Tips for Improving Grammar

1. Visit the Online Writing Lab website, which is sponsored by Purdue University, at http://owl.english.purdue.edu. This site provides you with an excellent overview of syntax, writing style, and strategy. It also has helpful and lengthy review sections that include multiple-choice "Test Your Knowledge" quizzes, which provide immediate answers to the questions.

2. It's beneficial to read the entire passage first to determine its intended meaning BEFORE you attempt to answer any questions. Doing so provides you with key insight into a passage's syntax (especially verb tense, subject-verb agreement, modifier placement, writing style, and punctuation).

3. When you answer a question, use the "Process-of-Elimination Method" to determine the best answer. Try each of the four answers and determine which one BEST fits with the meaning of the paragraph. Find the BEST answer. Chances are that the BEST answer is the CORRECT answer.

Test Your Knowledge: Grammar

1. A(n) _____ reflects a person, place, or thing.
   a) Noun
   b) Adjective
   c) Verb
   d) Conjunction

2. A(n) _____ expresses emotion.
   a) Pronoun
   b) Adverb
   c) Preposition
   d) Interjection

3. A _____ is a group of words that has a subject committing an action and a predicate.
   a) Clause
   b) Predicate
   c) Phrase
   d) Subject

4. A _____ is a group of words that does not have a subject committing an action.
   a) Clause
   b) Predicate
   c) Phrase
   d) Subject

5. *The man was short the woman was shorter.* This sentence has which of the following errors?
   a) Subject-verb agreement
   b) Comma splice
   c) Run-on
   d) None of the above

6. *The mother and daughter knew she danced well.* This sentence has which of the following errors?
   a) Unclear or vague pronoun reference
   b) Misplaced modifier
   c) Preposition at the end of a sentence
   d) None of the above

7. *The chairman made his decision.* This sentence has which of the following errors?
   a) Cliché
   b) Euphemism
   c) Sexist language
   d) None of the above

8. Which of the following sentences uses *affect/effect* correctly?
    a) The affect of the medication is overwhelming.
    b) The nurse's workload effected her performance.
    c) The effect of care was relieving.
    d) None of the above.

9. Which of the following sentences uses *amount/number* correctly?
    a) The amount of people in the hospital was overwhelming.
    b) There was a large number of water in the cooler.
    c) There is a great number of pages in the documentation.
    d) None of the above.

10. A(n) _____ is a clause that expresses a complete thought and can stand as its own sentence.
    a) Independent clause
    b) Dependent clause
    c) Compound sentence
    d) None of the above

11. A(n) _____ sentence reflects a statement.
    a) Exclamatory
    b) Interrogative
    c) Imperative
    d) Declarative

12. A _____ is a form of a verb that varies depending on the sentence in which it's used.
    a) Participle
    b) Phrase
    c) Predicate
    d) None of the above

Test Your Knowledge: Grammar—Answers

1. a)

2. d)

3. a)

4. c)

5. c)

6. a)

7. c)

8. c)

9. c)

10. a)

11. d)

12. a)

Chapter 4: Vocabulary

Communication is one of the most important aspects of the healthcare industry. Not only must you speak clearly to doctors and other healthcare professionals, but you must also write clearly for documentation purposes. On a daily basis, healthcare personnel use specific healthcare terminology as well as general terms within a medical context. It is crucial that you know both kinds of terms and how to use them in your daily communication.

The HESI vocabulary section will consist of the following types of questions: select the correct definition of the term, match the stated definition to the correct term, infer the definition of the term from its use in a sentence, select the term that will make the sentence grammatically correct, select the correct synonym of the term, identify the incorrectly spelled term, and select the correct order of the terms to be used in the sentence structure.

The words listed below include both specific and general terms you are likely to encounter on the HESI exam.

Abrupt- changing or terminating suddenly

Abstain- refrain

Access- means of approach or admission

Accountable- liable or responsible

Adhere- hold closely to an idea or course; be devoted

Adverse- harmful to one's interests; unfortunate

Affect- produce an affect or change on; influence

Annual- occurring or returning once a year

Apply- bring into physical contact; lay on; bring into operation

Audible- loud enough to be heard

Bilateral- having two sides

Cardiac- pertaining to the heart

Cast- a molded protective device used to support broken bones

Cavity- any hollow place or space

Cease- stop doing an action; discontinue

Compensatory- making up for; offsetting; paying for

Complication- something intricate, involved, or aggravating

Comply- acquiesce in another's wish, command, etc.

Concave- with an outline or surface curved like the inside of a ball; curved inward

Concise- brief and compact

Consistency- state of being congruous; conforming to regular patterns, habits, principles, etc.

Constrict- cause to shrink; cramp; crush

Contingent- depending on something not certain; conditional

Contour- the outline of a figure or shape

Contract- legal or business agreement; acquire a habit or disease

Contraindication- discouragement of the use of a treatment

Defecate- have a bowel movement

Deficit- shortage; excess of liabilities over assets

Depress- weaken; sadden

Depth- deepness; distance measured downward, inward, or backward

Deteriorating- growing worse; reducing in worth; impairing

Device- a gadget; a mechanical apparatus

Diagnosis- analysis of a present condition

Diameter- a line dividing a circle into halves; its length

Dilate- expand; make larger; distend

Dilute- weaken by a mixture of water or other liquid; reduce in strength

Discrete- separate; discontinuous

Distended- dilated; expanded; swollen

Dysfunction- impaired functioning

Elevate- raise; lift up

Endogenous- something produced within the body

Exacerbate- make more bitter, angry, or violent; irritate or aggravate

Excess- the state of being more or too much; a surplus or remainder

Exogenous- something produced outside the body

Expand- increase in extent, bulk, or amount; spread or stretch out; unfold

Exposure- the state of being exposed or open to external environments

External- located outside of something and/or apart from something

Fatal- causing death or ruin

Fatigue- weariness from physical or mental exertion

Flaccid- soft; flabby

Flushed- suffused with color; washed out with a copious flow of water

Gaping- to be open; to have a break in continuity

Gastrointestinal- pertaining to the stomach and intestines

Gender- the classification of masculine or feminine

Hematologic- dealing with the blood

Hydration- the act of meeting body fluid demands

Hygiene- the science that deals with the preservation of health

Impaired- made worse; damaged; weakened

Impending- the point of occurring; imminent

Incidence- frequency or range of occurrence; extent of effects

Infection- tainted with germs or disease

Inflamed- condition in which the body is inflicted with heat, swelling, and redness

Ingest- take into the body for digestion

Initiate- set going; begin; originate

Insidious- operating stealthily with evil effect; deceitful; treacherous

Intact- remaining uninjured, unimpaired, whole, or complete

Internal- situated within something; enclosed; inside

Invasive- being intrusive or encroaching upon

Labile- apt to lapse or err; unstable

Laceration- a rough tear; an affliction

Latent- hidden; dormant; undeveloped

Lethargic- not wanting to move; sluggish

Manifestation- a demonstration or display

Musculoskeletal- pertaining to muscles and the skeleton

Neurologic- dealing with the nervous system

Neurovascular- pertaining to the nervous system and blood vessels

Nutrient- something affording nutrition

Occluded- shut in or out; closed; absorbed

Ominous- foretelling disaster; threatening

Ongoing- continuous; constant

Oral- spoken, not written; pertaining to the mouth

Overt- plain to the view; open

Parameter- a variable quantity whose values depend on the special case

Paroxysmal- having to do with a spasm or violent outburst

Patent- open for all to read; plain; obvious

Pathogenic- causing disease

Pathology- the science of the nature and origin of disease

Posterior- located in the back or rear

Potent- wielding power; strong; effective

Potential- possible; possibility

Precaution- an act done in advance to assure safety or benefit; prudent foresight

Precipitous- over-hasty; rash; uncontrolled

Predispose- give a tendency or inclination to; dispose in advance

Preexisting- already in place; already occurring

Primary- first; earliest; most important

Priority- right of precedence; order of importance

Prognosis- a forecast

Rationale- rational basis for something; justification

Recur- appear again; return

Renal- pertaining to the kidneys

Respiration- breathing

Restrict- attach limitations to; restrain

Retain- hold or keep in possession, use, or practice

Site- location

Status- relative standing; position; condition

Strict- precise; exacting; severe

Sublingual- beneath the tongue

Supplement- an addition to something substantially completed; to add to

Suppress- restrain; abolish; repress

Symmetric- similar proportion in the size or shape of something

Symptom- a sign or indication of a problem or disease

Syndrome- a set of symptoms that characterize a certain disease or condition

Therapeutic- pertaining to the curing of disease; having remedial effect

Transdermal- passing through the skin

Transmission- the act or result of sending something along or onward to a recipient or destination

Trauma- a bodily injury or mental shock

Triage- the act of sorting or categorizing conditions and diseases in preparation for treatment

Untoward- unfavorable; troublesome

Urinate- discharge urine

Vascular- pertaining to bodily ducts that convey fluid

Verbal- expressed in words; oral, not written

Virus- an agent of infection

Vital- pertaining to life; alive; essential to existence or well-being

Void- empty; evacuate

Volume- a space filled by a fluid

Abate- become less in amount or intensity

Abdicate- to give up or leave

Abbreviate- to shorten or abridge

Abstain- choose to avoid or not participate

Adversity- a state of burden or hardship

Anecdote- a short story or account of an event

Assiduous- very careful and hardworking

Benevolent- showing sympathy, understanding, and generosity

Bias- an unfair preference or dislike of something

Boisterous- rough; rowdy; unruly

Brazen- bold or unrestrained by normal standards

Brusque- attitude of shortness or rudeness; gruff

Capacious- large in size or capacity

Circuitous- lengthy due to being indirect or roundabout

Collaborate- work together on a common project

Collateral- adjoining or accompanying

Compassion- awareness and sympathy for the suffering of others

Compromise- an accommodation in which both sides make concessions

Condescending- an attitude of superiority or being snobby toward others

Conditional- dependent on something else being done

Copious- abundant and plentiful

Concise- brief; condensed

Deleterious- harmful or deadly to living things

Deter- to prevent or discourage

Digression- a deviation or detour from the central topic or focus

Diligent- persistent and hardworking

Disdain- lack of respect or intense dislike

Empathy- understanding of another's feelings

Enhance- to improve; to increase clarity

Enervating- causing debilitation or weakness

Ephemeral- lasting only for a short period of time

Exasperate- worsen, make angry, or frustrate

Exemplary- worthy of imitation; setting the example

Extenuating- diminish the seriousness of something

Fortitude- strength and endurance during a difficult situation

Fortuitous- occurring by happy chance

Garble- confusing, not understandable

Hypothesis- a theory that has not yet been tested or investigated

Hyperbole- exaggerating; making something more than it is

Impetuous- undue haste without thought of consequences

Imminent- very likely to happen

Incompatible- unable to be or work together

Inconsequential- something without importance or significance

Inevitable- impossible to avoid or prevent from happening

Integrity- doing what is right, honest, or decent

Intuitive- to know by instinct alone

Innocuous- harmless

Longevity- having a long life

Languid- tired and slow

Novice- a beginner; inexperienced

Paradox- appearing conflicting or contradictory

Pragmatic- concerned with practical matters and results

Precocious- showing advanced development or maturity at an early age

Procrastinate- to postpone doing something that must be done

Prudent- careful and sensible; using good judgment

Resilient- quick to recover

Sagacity- sound knowledge, judgment, and foresight

Scrutinize- examine closely and carefully

Subtle- understated, not obvious

Superficial- shallow in character and attitude; only concerned with things on the surface

Superfluous- more than is needed, desired, or necessary

Tactful- showing concern to not offend others

Tenacious- determined without change or doubt from the plan

Terse- to the point; concise

Transient- lasting for only a short time or duration

Trite- dull; common

Venerable- worthy of respect because of wisdom or age

Venerate- to regard with much respect

Wary- to be cautious or suspicious

Test Your Knowledge: Vocabulary

Select the correct definition of the underlined term.

1. The medication had an <u>adverse</u> effect.
    a) Harmful
    b) Beneficial
    c) Limiting
    d) None of the above

2. The documentation was <u>concise</u>.
    a) Long
    b) Short
    c) Irrelevant
    d) None of the above

3. When assessing the patient, the nurse found several areas that had undergone <u>trauma</u>.
    a) Injury
    b) Shock
    c) Both A and B
    d) Neither A nor B

4. Before surgery, the patient had to <u>void</u> his bladder.
    a) Empty
    b) Fill
    c) Check
    d) None of the above

Match the definition in the sentence to the correct term.

5. The number of surgeries was <u>more than necessary</u>.
    a) Contraindicated
    b) Excessive
    c) Invasive
    d) None of the above

6. The patient was too <u>weakened and damaged</u> to drive.
    a) Assiduous
    b) Prudent
    c) Impaired
    d) None of the above

Select the correct synonym of the underlined term.

7. The <u>neurologic</u> assessment was completed before the diagnosis.
    a) Nervous system
    b) Skeletal system
    c) Gastrointestinal system
    d) None of the above

8. The <u>main</u> nurse had just finished caring for the patient.
    a) Primary
    b) Secondary
    c) Priority
    d) None of the above

Select the term that will make the sentence grammatically correct.

9. Nurses avoid _____ a patient as often as possible.
    a) Instructing
    b) Releasing
    c) Restricting
    d) None of the above

10. The patient showed many _____ of Down's syndrome.
    a) Symptoms
    b) Rejections
    c) Contraindications
    d) None of the above

Test Your Knowledge: Vocabulary—Answers

1. a)

2. b)

3. c)

4. a)

5. b)

6. c)

7. a)

8. a)

9. c)

10. a)

Chapter 5: Biology

BASICS OF LIFE

We began learning the difference between living (**animate**) beings and nonliving (**inanimate**) objects from an early age. Living organisms and inanimate objects are all composed of **atoms** from elements. Those atoms are arranged into groups called **molecules**, which serve as the building blocks of everything in existence (as we know it). Molecular interactions are what determine whether something is classified as animate or inanimate. The following is a list of the most commonly-found elements found in the molecules of animate beings:

- Oxygen
- Chlorine
- Carbon
- Nitrogen
- Sodium
- Calcium
- Magnesium
- Phosphorous
- Iodine
- Iron
- Sulfur
- Hydrogen
- Potassium

Another way to describe living and nonliving things is through the terms **organic** and **inorganic.**

- **Organic molecules** are from living organisms. Organic molecules contain **carbon-hydrogen bonds**.
- **Inorganic molecules** come from non-living resources. They do not contain carbon-hydrogen bonds.

There are four major classes of organic molecules:

1. **Carbohydrates**
2. **Lipids**
3. **Proteins**
4. **Nucleic acids**.

Carbohydrates

Carbohydrates consist of only hydrogen, oxygen, and carbon atoms. They are the most abundant single class of organic substances found in nature. Carbohydrate molecules provide many basic necessities such as: fiber, vitamins, and minerals; structural components for organisms, especially plants; and, perhaps most importantly, energy. Our bodies break down carbohydrates to make **glucose**: a sugar used to produce that energy which our bodies need in order to operate. Brain cells are exclusively dependent upon a constant source of glucose molecules.

There are two kinds of carbohydrates: simple and complex.

> **Simple carbohydrates** can be absorbed directly through the cell, and therefore enter the blood stream very quickly. We consume simple carbohydrates in dairy products, fruits, and other sugary foods.

> **Complex carbohydrates** consist of a chain of simple sugars which, over time, our bodies break down into simple sugars (which are also referred to as stored energy.) **Glycogen** is the storage form of glucose in human and animal cells. Complex carbohydrates come from starches like cereal, bread, beans, potatoes, and starchy vegetables.

Lipids

Lipids, commonly known as fats, are molecules with two functions:

1. They are stored as an energy reserve.
2. They provide a protective cushion for vital organs.

In addition to those two functions, lipids also combine with other molecules to form essential compounds, such as **phospholipids,** which form the membranes around cells. Lipids also combine with other molecules to create naturally-occurring **steroid** hormones, like the hormones estrogen and testosterone.

Proteins

Proteins are large molecules which our bodies' cells need in order to function properly. Consisting of **amino acids,** proteins aid in maintaining and creating many aspects of our cells: cellular structure, function, and regulation, to name a few. Proteins also work as neurotransmitters and carriers of oxygen in the blood (hemoglobin).

Without protein, our tissues and organs could not exist. Our muscles bones, skin, and many other parts of the body contain significant amounts of protein. **Enzymes**, hormones, and antibodies are proteins.

Enzymes
When heat is applied, chemical reactions are typically sped up. However, the amount of heat required to speed up reactions could be potentially harmful (even fatal) to living organisms. Instead, our bodies use molecules called enzymes to bring reactants closer together, causing them to form a new compound. Thus, the whole reaction rate is increased without heat. Even better – the enzymes are not consumed during the reaction process, and can therefore be used reused. This makes them an important biochemical part of both photosynthesis and respiration.

Nucleic Acid

Nucleic acids are large molecules made up of smaller molecules called **nucleotides. DNA** (deoxyribonucleic acid) transports and transmits genetic information. As you can tell from the name, DNA is a nucleic acid. Since nucleotides make up nucleic acids, they are considered the basis of reproduction and progression.

Test Your Knowledge: Basics of Life

1. Life depends upon:
    a) The bond energy in molecules.
    b) The energy of protons.
    c) The energy of electrons.
    d) The energy of neutrons.

2. Which of the following elements is **NOT** found in carbohydrates?
    a) Carbon.
    b) Hydrogen.
    c) Oxygen.
    d) Sulfur.

3. Which of the following is a carbohydrate molecule?
    a) Amino acid.
    b) Glycogen.
    c) Sugar.
    d) Lipid.

4. Lipids are commonly known as:
    a) Fat.
    b) Sugar.
    c) Enzymes.
    d) Protein.

5. Proteins are composed of:
    a) Nucleic acids.
    b) Amino acids.
    c) Hormones.
    d) Lipids.

Test Your Knowledge: Basics of Life – Answers

1. a)
2. d)
3. c)
4. a)
5. b)

CELLULAR RESPIRATION

As you can imagine, there are a great deal of processes which require energy: breathing, blood circulation, body temperature control, muscle usage, digestion, brain and nerve functioning are all only a few examples. You can refer to all of the body's physical and chemical processes which convert or use energy as **metabolism**.

All living things in the world, including plants, require energy in order to maintain their metabolisms. Initially, that energy is consumed through food. That energy is processed in plants and animals through **photosynthesis** (for plants) and **respiration** (for animals). **Cellular respiration** produces the actual energy molecules known as **ATP** (Adenosine Tri-Phosphate) molecules.

Plants use ATP during **photosynthesis** for producing glucose, which is then broken down during cellular respiration. This cycle continuously repeats itself throughout the life of the plant.

Photosynthesis: Plants, as well as some Protists and Monerans, can use light energy to bind together small molecules from the environment. These newly-bound molecules are then used as fuel to make more energy. This process is called photosynthesis, and one of its byproducts is none other than oxygen. Most organisms, including plants, require oxygen to fuel the biochemical reactions of metabolism.

You can see in the following equation that plants use the energy taken from light to turn carbon dioxide and water – the small molecules from their environment – into glucose and oxygen.

The photosynthesis equation:

$$CO_2 + H_2O \xrightarrow{\text{Light}} C_6H_{12}O_6 + O_2$$

Carbon Dioxide   Water   Glucose (sugar)   Oxygen

Chlorophyll

In order for photosynthesis to occur, however, plants require a specific molecule to capture sunlight. This molecule is called **chlorophyll**. When chlorophyll absorbs sunlight, one of its electrons is stimulated into a higher energy state. This higher-energy electron then passes that energy onto other electrons in other molecules, creating a chain that eventually results in glucose. Chlorophyll absorbs red and blue light, but not green; green light is reflected off of plants, which is why plants appear green to us. It's important to note that chlorophyll is absolutely necessary to the photosynthesis process in plants –if it photosynthesizes, it will have chlorophyll.

The really fascinating aspect of photosynthesis is that raw sunlight energy is a very nonliving thing; however, it is still absorbed by plants to form the chemical bonds between simple inanimate compounds. This produces organic sugar, which is the chemical basis for the formation of all living compounds. Isn't it amazing? Something nonliving is essential to the creation of all living things!

Respiration

Respiration is the metabolic opposite of photosynthesis. There are two types of respiration: **aerobic** (which uses oxygen) and **anaerobic** (which occurs without the use of oxygen).

You may be confused at thinking of the word "respiration" in this way, since many people use respiration to refer to the process of breathing. However, in biology, breathing is thought of as **inspiration** (inhaling) and **expiration** (exhalation); whereas **respiration** is the metabolic, chemical reaction supporting these processes. Both plants and animals produce carbon dioxide through respiration.

Aerobic respiration is the reaction which uses enzymes to combine oxygen with organic matter (food). This yields carbon dioxide, water, and energy.

The respiration equation looks like this:

Enzymes
$$C6H12O6 + 6O2 \longrightarrow 7\ 6CO2 + 6H2O + energy$$

If you look back the equation for photosynthesis, you will see that respiration is almost the same equation, only it goes in the opposite direction. (Photosynthesis uses carbon dioxide and water, with the help of energy, to create oxygen and glucose. Respiration uses oxygen and glucose, with the help of enzymes, to create carbon dioxide, water, and energy.)

Anaerobic respiration is respiration that occurs WITHOUT the use of oxygen. It produces less energy than aerobic respiration produces, yielding only two molecules of ATP per glucose molecule Aerobic respiration produces 38 ATP per glucose molecule.

So, plants convert energy into matter and release oxygen gas – animals then absorb this oxygen gas in order to run their own metabolic reaction and, in the process, release carbon dioxide. That carbon dioxide is then absorbed by plants in the photosynthetic conversion of energy into matter. Everything comes full circle! This is called a **metabolic cycle.**

Test Your Knowledge: Cellular Respiration

1. Which of the following is **NOT** true of enzymes?
    a) Enzymes are lipid molecules.
    b) Enzymes are not consumed in a biochemical reaction.
    c) Enzymes are important in photosynthesis and respiration.
    d) Enzymes speed up reactions and make them more efficient.

2. Plants appear green because chlorophyll:
    a) Absorbs green light.
    b) Reflects red light.
    c) Absorbs blue light.
    d) Reflects green light.

3. Photosynthesis is the opposite of:
    a) Enzymatic hydrolysis.
    b) Protein synthesis.
    c) Respiration.
    d) Reproduction.

4. The compound that absorbs light energy during photosynthesis is:
    a) Chloroform.
    b) Chlorofluorocarbon.
    c) Chlorinated biphenyls.
    d) Chlorophyll.

5. What is the name of the sugar molecule produced during photosynthesis?
    a) Chlorophyll.
    b) Glycogen.
    c) Glucose.
    d) Fructose.

Test Your Knowledge: Cellular Respiration – Answers

1. a)
2. d)
3. c)
4. d)
5. c)

CLASSIFICATION OF ORGANISMS

All of Earth's organisms have characteristics which distinguish them from one another. Scientists have developed systems to organize and classify all of Earth's organisms based on those characteristics.

Kingdoms

Through the process of evolution, organisms on Earth have developed into many diverse forms, which have complex relationships. Scientists have organized life into five large groups called **kingdoms**. Each kingdom contains those organisms that share significant characteristics distinguishing them from organisms in other kingdoms. These five kingdoms are named as follows:

1. **Animalia**
2. **Plantae**
3. **Fungi**
4. **Protista**
5. **Monera**

Kingdom Animalia

This kingdom contains multicellular organisms multicellular, or those known as complex organisms. These organisms are generically called **heterotrophs**, which means that they must eat preexisting organic matter (either plants or other animals) in order to sustain themselves.

Those heterotrophs which eat only plants are called **herbivores** (from "herbo," meaning "herb" or "plant"); those that kill and eat other animals for food are called **carnivores** (from "carno," meaning "flesh" or "meat"); and still other animals eat both plants *and* other animals – they are called **omnivores** (from "omnis," which means "all").

Those organisms in the Animal Kingdom have nervous tissue which has developed into nervous systems and brains; they are also able to move from place to place using muscular systems. The Animal Kingdom is divided into two groups: **vertebrates** (with backbones) and **invertebrates** (without backbones).

Kingdom Plantae

As you can guess from its name, the Plant Kingdom contains all plant-based life. Plants are multicellular organisms that use chlorophyll, which is held in specialized cellular structures called **chloroplasts,** to capture sunlight energy. Remember: photosynthesis! They then convert that sunlight energy into organic matter: their food. Because of this, most plants are referred to as **autotrophs** (self-feeders). There are a few organisms included in the Plant Kingdom which are not multicellular – certain types of algae which, while not multicellular, have cells with a nucleus. These algae also contain chlorophyll.

Except for algae, most plants are divided into one of two groups: **vascular plants** (most crops, trees, and flowering plants) and **nonvascular plants** (mosses). Vascular plants have specialized tissue that allows them to transport water and nutrients from their roots, to their leaves, and back again – even when the plant is several hundred feet tall. Nonvascular plants cannot do this, and therefore remain very small in size. Vascular plants are able to grow in both wet and dry environments; whereas nonvascular plants, since they are unable to transport water, are usually found only in wet, marshy areas.

Kingdom Fungi

The Fungi Kingdom contains organisms that share some similarities with plants, but also have other characteristics that make them more animal-like. For example, they resemble animals in that they lack chlorophyll – so they can't perform photosynthesis. This means that they don't produce their own food and are therefore heterotrophs.

However, they resemble plants in that they reproduce by spores; they also resemble plants in appearance. The bodies of fungi are made of filaments called **hyphae**, which in turn create the tissue **mycelium.** The most well-known examples of organisms in this Kingdom are mushrooms, yeasts, and molds. Fungi are very common and benefit other organisms, including humans.

Kingdom Protista

This kingdom includes single-celled organisms that contain a nucleus as part of their structure. They are considered a simple cell, but still contain multiple structures and accomplish many functions. This Kingdom includes organisms such as paramecium, amoeba, and slime molds. They often move around using hair-like structures called *cilia* or *flagellums.*

Kingdom Monera

This kingdom contains only bacteria. All of these organisms are single-celled and do not have a nucleus. They have only one chromosome, which is used to transfer genetic information. Sometimes they can also transmit genetic information using small structures called **plasmids.** Like organisms in the Protista Kingdom, they use flagella to move. Bacteria usually reproduce asexually.

There are more forms of bacteria than any other organism on Earth. Some bacteria are beneficial to us, like the ones found in yogurt; others can cause us to get sick such as the bacteria *E. coli.*

KINGDOM	DESCRIPTION	EXAMPLES
Animalia	Multi-celled; parasites; prey; consumers; can be herbivorous, carnivorous, or omnivorous	Sponges, worms, insects, fish, mammals, reptiles, birds, humans
Plantae	Multi-celled; autotrophs; mostly producers	Ferns, angiosperms, gymnosperms, mosses
Fungi	Can be single or multi-celled; decomposers; parasites; absorb food; asexual; consumers	Mushrooms, mildew, molds, yeast
Protista	Single or multi-celled; absorb food; both producers and consumers	Plankton, algae, amoeba, protozoans
Monera	Single-celled or a colony of single-cells; decomposers and parasites; move in water; are both producers and consumers	Bacteria, blue-green algae

Levels of Classification

Kingdom groupings are not very specific. They contain organisms defined by broad characteristics, and which may not seem similar at all. For example, worms belong in Kingdom Animalia – but then, so do birds. These two organisms are very different, despite sharing the necessary traits to make it into the animal kingdom. Therefore, to further distinguish different organisms, we have multiple levels of classification, which gradually become more specific until we finally reach the actual organism.

We generally start out by grouping organisms into the appropriate kingdom. Within each kingdom, we have other subdivisions: **Phylum, Class, Order, Family, Genus, and Species.** (In some cases, "Species" can be further narrowed down into "Sub-Species.")

As we move down the chain, characteristics become more specific, and the number of organisms in each group decreases. For an example, let's try to classify a grizzly bear. The chart would go as follows:

Kingdom - insect, fish, bird, pig, dog, bear

Phylum - fish, bird, pig, dog, bear

Class - pig, dog, bear

Order - dog, bear

Family - panda, brown, grizzly

Genus - brown, grizzly

Species - grizzly

Here is an easy way to remember the order of terms used in this classification scheme:

Kings **P**lay **C**ards **O**n **F**riday, **G**enerally **S**peaking.

Kingdom, **P**hylum, **C**lass, **O**rder, **F**amily, **G**enus, **S**pecies

Binomial Nomenclature

Organisms can be positively identified by two Latin words. Therefore, the organism naming system is referred to as a binomial nomenclature ("binomial" referring to the number two, and "nomenclature" referring to a title or name). Previously-used words help illustrate where the organism fits into the whole scheme, but it is only the last two, the genus and species, that specifically name an organism. Both are written in italics. The genus is always capitalized, but the species name is written lowercase.

Grizzly bears fall underneath the genus *Ursus*, species *arctos*, and sub-species *horribilis*. Therefore, the scientific name of the grizzly bear would be *Ursus arctos horribilis*. *Canis familiaris* is the scientific name for a common dog, *Felis domesticus* is a common cat, and humans are *Homo sapiens*.

Test Your Knowledge: Classification of Organisms

1. Which feature distinguishes those organisms in Kingdom Monera from those in other kingdoms? Organisms in Kingdom Monera:
   a) Contain specialized organelles.
   b) Contain a nucleus.
   c) Contain chloroplasts.
   d) Lack a nucleus.

2. Which of the following has the classification levels in the correct order, from most general to most specific?
   a) Kingdom, Phylum, Class, Order, Family, Genus, Species.
   b) Order, Family, Genus, Species, Class, Phylum, Kingdom.
   c) Species, Genus, Family, Order, Class, Phylum, Kingdom.
   d) Kingdom, Phylum, Class, Species, Genus, Family, Order.

3. The _____ contains organisms with both plant-and-animal-like characteristics?
   a) Animal Kingdom.
   b) Plant Kingdom.
   c) Fungi Kingdom.
   d) Monera Kingdom.

4. Which of the following statements is true about the binomial nomenclature system of classification?
   a) The genus and species names describe a specific organism.
   b) The category of kingdom is very specific.
   c) The category of species is very broad.
   d) Three names are needed to correctly specify a particular organism.

5. Which of the following kingdom's members are multicellular AND autotrophic?
   a) Fungi.
   b) Animalia.
   c) Protista.
   d) Plantae.

Test Your Knowledge: Classification of Organisms – Answers

1. d)

2. a)

3. c)

4. a)

5. d)

CELLS, TISSUES, AND ORGANS

All organisms are composed of microscopic cells, although the type and number of cells may vary. A cell is the minimum amount of organized living matter that is complex enough to carry out the functions of life. This section will briefly review both animal and plant cells, noting their basic similarities and differences.

Cell Structure

Around the cell is the **cell membrane**, which separates the living cell from the rest of the environment and regulates the comings and goings of molecules within the cell. Because the cell membrane allows some molecules to pass through while blocking others, it is considered **semipermeable.** Each cell's membrane communicates and interacts with the membranes of other cells. In additional to a cell membrane, *plants* also have a **cell wall** which is necessary for structural support and protection. Animal cells do not contain a cell wall.

Organelle

Cells are filled with a gelatin-like substance called **protoplasm** which contains various structures called **organelles**; called so because they act like small versions of organs. The diagram on the next page illustrates the basic organelles of both a plant and an animal cell. Pay attention to the differences and similarities between the two.

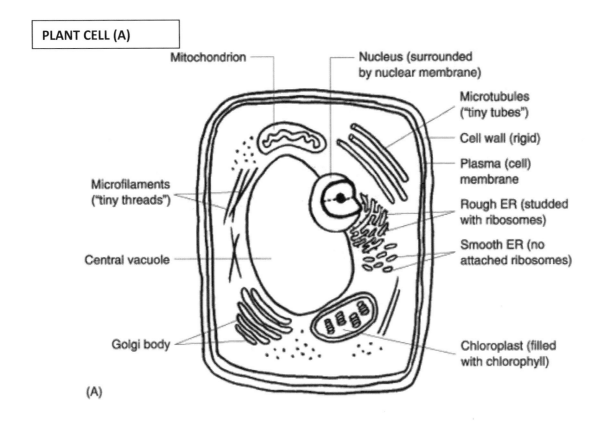

PLANT CELL (A)

Mitochondrion

Nucleus (surrounded by nuclear membrane)

Microtubules ("tiny tubes")

Cell wall (rigid)

Plasma (cell) membrane

Rough ER (studded with ribosomes)

Smooth ER (no attached ribosomes)

Microfilaments ("tiny threads")

Central vacuole

Golgi body

Chloroplast (filled with chlorophyll)

(A)

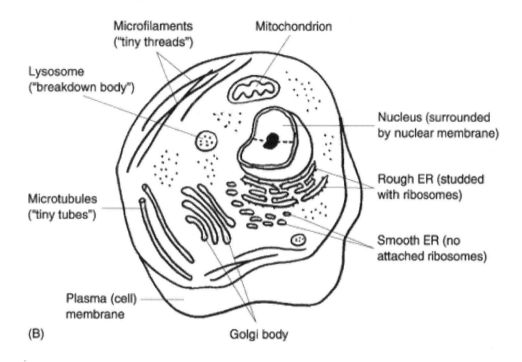

Microfilaments ("tiny threads")

Mitochondrion

Lysosome ("breakdown body")

Nucleus (surrounded by nuclear membrane)

Microtubules ("tiny tubes")

Rough ER (studded with ribosomes)

Smooth ER (no attached ribosomes)

Plasma (cell) membrane

(B)

Golgi body

Organelles (Defined)

Mitochondria are spherical or rod-shaped organelles which carry out the reactions of aerobic respiration. They are the power generators of both plant and animal cells, because they convert oxygen and nutrients into ATP, the chemical energy that powers the cell's metabolic activities.

Ribosomes are extremely tiny spheres that make proteins. These proteins are used either as enzymes or as support for other cell functions.

The **Golgi Apparatus** is essential to the production of polysaccharides (carbohydrates), and made up of a layered stack of flattened sacs.

The **Endoplasmic Reticulum** is important in the synthesis and packaging of proteins. It is a complex system of internal membranes, and is called either rough (when ribosomes are attached), or smooth (no ribosomes attached).

Chloroplasts are only found in plants. They contain the chlorophyll molecule necessary for photosynthesis.

The **Nucleus** controls all of the cell's functions, and contains the all-important genetic information, or DNA, of a cell.

Cellular Differentiation

Single-celled organisms have only one cell to carry out all of their required biochemical and structural functions. On the other hand, multi-celled organisms – except for very primitive ones (i.e. sponges) – have various groups of cells called **tissues** that each perform specific functions (**differentiation**).

There are four main types of tissues: **epithelial, connective, muscular,** and **nervous**.

Epithelial tissue is made up groups of flattened cells which are grouped tightly together to form a solid surface. Those cells are arranged in one or many layer(s) to form an external or internal covering of the body or organs. Epithelial tissue protects the body from injury and allows for the exchange of gases in the lungs and bronchial tubes. There's even a form of epithelial tissue that produces eggs and sperm, an organism's sex cells.

Connective tissue is made of cells which are surrounded by non-cellular material. For example, bones contain some cells, but they are also surrounded by a considerable amount of non-cellular, extracellular material.

Muscular tissue has the ability to contract. There are three types:

1. **Cardiac** tissue, found in the heart.

2. **Smooth** tissue, located in the walls of hollow internal structures such as blood vessels, the stomach, intestines, and urinary bladder.

3. **Skeletal** (or striated) tissue, found in the muscles.

Nervous tissue consists of cells called **neurons.** Neurons specialize in making many connections with and transmitting electrical impulses to each other. The brain, spinal cord, and peripheral nerves are all made of nervous tissue.

Organs and Organ Systems

As living organisms go through their life cycle, they grow and/or develop. Single-celled organisms grow and develop very rapidly; whereas complex, multi-celled organisms take much longer to progress. All organisms go through changes as they age. These changes involve the development of more complex functions, which in turn require groups of tissues to form larger units called **organs.** Here are some examples of organs:

1. **The heart** - Made of cardiac muscle and conjunctive tissue (conjunctive tissue makes up the valves), the heart pumps blood first to the lungs in order to pick up oxygen, then through the rest of the body to deliver the oxygen, and finally back to the lungs to start again.

2. **Roots** - A tree's are covered by an epidermis which is in turn made up of a protective tissue. They are also *composed* of tissue, which allows them to grow. The root organ also contains **conductive tissue** to absorb and transport water and nutrients to the rest of the plant.

Generally, in complex organisms like plants and animals, many organs are grouped together into **systems.** For example, many combinations of tissues make up the many organs which create the digestive system in animals. The organs in the digestive system consist of the mouth, the esophagus, the stomach, small and large intestines, the liver, the pancreas, and the gall bladder.

Test Your Knowledge: Cells, Tissues, and Organs

1. Which statement is true about Earth's organisms?
   a) All organisms are based on the cell as the basic unit of life.
   b) Protists are an exception to the cell theory and are not based on cells.
   c) Only single-celled organisms are based on cells.
   d) All organisms are based on tissues as the basic unit of life.

2. What organelle produces the cell's energy source?
   a) Chloroplast.
   b) Nucleus.
   c) Mitochondrion.
   d) Endoplasmic reticulum.

3. The formation of tissue depends upon:
   a) Cell differentiation.
   b) Cell membranes.
   c) Cell death.
   d) Cell organelles.

4. Cardiac muscle is an example of what tissue?
   a) Smooth muscle.
   b) Nervous.
   c) Contractile.
   d) Connective.

5. Which organelle has two forms: rough and smooth?
   a) Mitochondrion.
   b) Golgi apparatus.
   c) Nucleus.
   d) Endoplasmic reticulum.

Test Your Knowledge: Cells, Tissues, and Organs – Answers

1. a)
2. c)
3. a)
4. c)
5. d)

HEREDITY

A duck's webbed feet, a tree whose leaves change color in the fall, and humans having backbones are all characteristics inherited from parent organisms. These inheritable characteristics are transmitted through **genes** and **chromosomes**. In sexual reproduction, each parent contributes half of his or her genes to the offspring.

Genes

Genes influence both what we look like on the outside and how we work on the inside. They contain the information that our bodies need to make the proteins in our bodies. Genes are made of DNA: a double helix (spiral) molecule that consists of two long, twisted strands of nucleic acids. Each of these strands are made of sugar and phosphate molecules, and are connected by pairs of chemicals called **nitrogenous bases** (just bases, for short). There are four types of bases:

1. **Adenine (A)**
2. **Thymine (T)**
3. **Guanine (G)**
4. **Cytosine (C)**

These bases link in a very specific way: **A** always pairs with **T**, and **C** always pairs with **G**.

A gene is a piece of DNA that codes for a specific protein. Each gene contains the information necessary to produce a single trait in an organism, and each gene is different from any other. For example, one gene will code for the protein insulin, and another will code for hair. For any trait, we inherit one gene from our father and one from our mother. Human beings have 20,000 to 25,000 genes, yet those genes only account for about 3% of our DNA.

Alternate forms of the same gene are called **alleles**. When the alleles are identical, the individual is **homozygous** for that trait. When the alleles are different, the individual is **heterozygous** for that trait.

For example, a child may have red hair because she inherited two identical red color genes from each parent; that would make her homozygous for red hair. However, a second child may have brown hair because he inherited different hair color genes from each parent; this would make him heterozygous for brown hair. When genes exist in a heterozygous pairing, usually one is expressed over the other. The gene which is expressed is **dominant**. The unexpressed gene is called **recessive**.

If you took the DNA from all the cells in your body and lined it up, end to end, it would form a (very thin!) strand 6000 million miles long! DNA molecules, and their important genetic material, are tightly packed around proteins called **histones** to make structures called **chromosomes**. Human beings have 23 pairs of chromosomes in every cell, for 46 chromosomes in total. The sex chromosomes determine whether you are a boy (XY) or a girl (XX). The other chromosomes are called autosomes.

Patterns of Inheritance

Biologists refer to the genetic makeup of an organism as its **genotype**. However, the collection of physical characteristics that result from the action of genes is called an organism's **phenotype**. You can remember this differentiation by looking at the beginning of each word: *geno*type is *gen*etic, and *pheno*type is *phy*sical. Patterns of inheritance can produce surprising results, because the genotype determines the phenotype.

Test Your Knowledge: Heredity

1. On paired chromosomes, two identical alleles are called:
    a) Heterozygous.
    b) Homozygous.
    c) Tetrad.
    d) Binomial.

2. The physical characteristics of an organism are known as its:
    a) Chromosomes.
    b) Genotype.
    c) DNA.
    d) Phenotype.

3. Which of the following is **NOT** a nucleotide found in DNA?
    a) Uracil.
    b) Guanine.
    c) Cytosine.
    d) Thymine.

4. The genotype describes an organism's:
    a) Appearance.
    b) Genetic code.
    c) Type of DNA.
    d) Eye color only.

5. The shape of the DNA molecule is a:
    a) Single spiral.
    b) Double spiral.
    c) Straight chain.
    d) Bent chain.

Test Your Knowledge: Heredity – Answers

1. **b)**
2. **d)**
3. **a)**
4. **b)**
5. **b)**

NUCLEIC ACIDS & DNA STRUCTURE

Nucleic acids are long chain, polymeric molecules that are known to be essential to life on Earth. They are responsible for encoding protein sequences which are necessary for life to function. there are two main types of nucleic acid: DNA – deoxyribonucleic acid, and RNA – ribonucleic acid. The primary difference between these two are the structure of their sugar backbone, and the types of nucleotide bases that are present.

DNA – DNA is the primary code of life. It is a double stranded helix. Each strand consists of a sugar backbone of deoxyribose, and associated nucleotide bases. The bases that are seen in DNA are guanine, adenine, thymine, and cytosine. They are represented respectively by the single letter codes G, A, T, and C. The nucleotide bases are complementary to one another. A & T will form a hydrogen bond between one another, and G and C will form a bond. The basic structure of these four compounds is seen below:

| Guanine | Adenine | Thymine | Cytosine |

Guanine and adenine are pyrimidine compounds, which have two rings, and thymine and cytosine are purine compounds, which have just a single ring. These nucleic acids form long sequences which are called genes. Genes are sequences of DNA that can be read by an enzyme and ribosome complex in order to produce proteins.

RNA – RNA is a single stranded nucleic acid strand that can codes for an amino acid sequence. In some species, such as viruses, RNA is the only form of genetic material that exists. In most species, both DNA and RNA are used. The sugar backbone of RNA is ribose, which is 5 carbon sugar. The nucleotides that are present in RNA are similar to DNA, with one exception. Instead of thymine, the RNA structure contains uracil, seen below:

RNA can be produced from DNA using the enzyme RNA polymerase, which binds to a DNA strand to produce a complementary copy.

Practice Problems for Nucleic Acids & DNA Structure

1. Which of the following is true about DNA?
   a) All living species have DNA
   b) DNA and RNA have the same sugar backbone
   c) DNA is only contained in your sex cells
   d) Humans have more DNA and chromosomes than any other species

2. Which of the following molecules is a pyrimidine?
   a) Uracil
   b) Thymine
   c) Cytosine
   d) Guanine

3. A scientist extracts some DNA from a plant and finds that the nucleic acid composition is as follows: 21% A, 29% G, 29% C, and 21% T. This is:
   a) A strand of RNA
   b) A single stranded DNA fragment
   c) A double stranded DNA fragment
   d) None of the above

4. Given the sequence ATGAACT, what is the correct complementary DNA sequence?
   a) GTACCGT
   b) TACTTGA
   c) TTACCGA
   d) ATGAATC

5. Given the sequence GCCATATG, what is the correct complementary RNA sequence?
   a) CGGUAUAC
   b) CGUTAUTC
   c) AGTCCATC
   d) CGGTATAC

Answer Key to Practice Problems
   1. A
   2. D
   3. C
   4. B
   5. A

MITOSIS & MEIOSIS

Mitosis and Meiosis are two forms of cell division in life. Mitosis is the process of a single cell splitting to form two new somatic cells. Somatic cells are any cell that is not a reproductive sex cell. Meiosis is a form of cell division in which half the DNA from a sex cell is enclosed into a gamete, such as sperm or an egg in humans. The cell product of Meiosis has half the DNA from before, and the two sex cells can be merged to form an embryo.

Mitosis

In mitosis, there are 5 major phases: Interphase, prophase, metaphase, anaphase, and telophase. These are the 5 phases the cell will go through to produce DNA and then split. The diagram below shows the basic process.

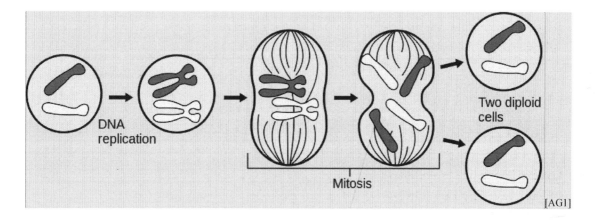

Interphase: In interphase, which is the growth phase, the cell has recently divided and is growing again. During this period of time, new proteins are being made as well as additional organelles. Additional DNA is also made during this phase.

Prophase: In this stage, the cell is preparing to divide. The DNA condenses into chromatin and forms into chromosomes. The centrioles within the cell migrate to opposite ends of the cell.

Metaphase: In metaphase, the centrioles have attached actin filaments to the individual chromosomes, and have started pulling them to opposite ends of the cell. The cell itself begins to elongate and stretch.

Anaphase: In anaphase, the chromosomes cleave, and there are now two sets of diploid chromosomes (represented in the figure as the 4th stage).

Telophase & Cytokinesis: The chromosomes are now on separate ends of the cell, and the cell membrane splits. Two new cells are now formed which are now both in interphase again.

The process of mitosis is important for growth in organisms, and is also how single celled organisms, such as bacteria and yeast, reproduce.

Meiosis

Meiosis only occurs in eukaryotes, and is a process necessary to produce sex cells for sexual reproduction. In short, meiosis takes random parts of chromosomes from the diploid (2n) set of chromosomes a parent has, and forms a haploid (1n) sex cell. As seen in the figure below, in the process of meiosis, homologous chromosomes are split into a total of 4 daughter nuclei.

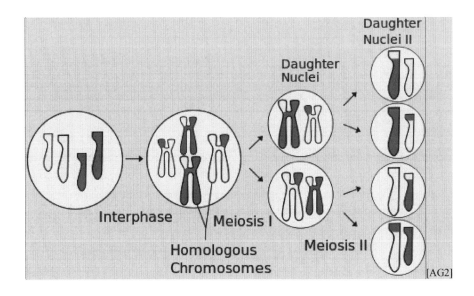

There are two major phases in meiosis: Meiosis I & Meisosi II.

Meiosis I – In the first stage of meiosis, the cell (in humans at least) starts with 23 pairs of chromosomes, or 46 total chromosomes. During Meiosis I, crossing over occurs. Crossing over is a process in which homologous (homologous means "same") chromosomes exchange parts with one another. The crossing over phenomenon is the primary generator of variation in species which use sexual reproduction.

After crossing over occurs, the cell splits into 2 daughter cells, each with a set of 23 chromosomes, but are now haploid. Each chromosome consists of a pair of sister chromatids.

Meiosis II – In Meiosis II, the process is essentially the same as mitosis, with sister chromatids being separated into a total of four cells. Each of these cells will contain one pair of sister chromatids. The sister chromatids in these now gametes will be able to fuse with another pair of sister chromatids from another sex cell to create an embryo.

Practice Problems for Mitosis & Meiosis

1. During which stage of mitosis is DNA created?
    a) Interphase
    b) Metaphase
    c) Telophase
    d) Anaphase

2. The centrioles are responsible for:
    a) Organizing the mitochondria in the cell
    b) Starting cell division
    c) Organizing the mitotic spindle
    d) Pulling apart the nuclear membrane

3. If a human cell undergoes mitosis, how many copies of each chromosome will be present in the each daughter cell?
    a) 1
    b) 2
    c) 3
    d) 4

4. A single cell undergoes mitosis every 20 minutes. How many cells will be present after 2 hours?
    a) 8
    b) 16
    c) 32
    d) 64

5. Which of the following is not true of *both* mitosis and meiosis?
    a) All daughter cells end up as diploid cells in both processes
    b) In both processes, 2 or more daughter cells are produced
    c) Both processes make use of centrioles
    d) Both processes can occur in eukaryotic cells

Answer Key to Practice Problems

1. A
2. C
3. B
4. D
5. A

DNA TRANSCRIPTION & TRANSLATION

DNA transcription and translation is the process through which the DNA code is "read" and forms a product protein. The protein then functions for a variety of different operations, including catalyzing reactions, acting as a channel in the cell membrane, or breaking down substances that are no longer useful in the cell. The transcription and translation pathway follows the basic steps seen in the figure below:

$$DNA \rightarrow RNA \rightarrow Ribosome + Nucleotides \rightarrow Protein$$

Step 1: DNA transcription: In the first step, called DNA transcription, a strand of DNA is copied by RNA polymerase into a strand of messenger RNA (mRNA). First, RNA polymerase, along with some promoter proteins, binds to DNA, unwinding it slightly. Then, RNA makes a copy of the DNA sequence using nucleotides, forming a strand of messenger RNA. The RNA is produced from the 3' end to the 5' end.

After the mRNA strand has been produced, the intron regions need to be removed. The intron regions are non-coding portions of DNA that don't "mean" anything. The introns are removed by a complex called the spliceosome, and the remaining exons (the coding regions), are spliced back together to get the final mRNA product.

Step 2: RNA translation: In the 2nd major step, the mRNA strand is carried to a ribosome. The majority of ribosomes are located on the endoplasmic reticulum in eukaryotic cells, although some ribosomes are free floating in the cytoplasm as well. The ribosome is a large complex of enzymes whose purpose is to read the mRNA and assemble a string of amino acids, which will later be folded into a protein.

The mRNA strand is read in sets of 3. Each set of 3 nucleotides, called a codon, in the mRNA strand represents an amino acid. A codon table and the represented amino acid is seen in the table below:

120

1st base	2nd base								3rd base
	U		C		A		G		
U	UUU	(Phe/F) Phenylalanine	UCU	(Ser/S) Serine	UAU	(Tyr/Y) Tyrosine	UGU	(Cys/C) Cysteine	U
	UUC		UCC		UAC		UGC		C
	UUA	(Leu/L) Leucine	UCA		UAA	Stop (Ochre)	UGA	Stop (Opal)	A
	UUG		UCG		UAG	Stop (Amber)	UGG	(Trp/W) Tryptophan	G
C	CUU	(Leu/L) Leucine	CCU	(Pro/P) Proline	CAU	(His/H) Histidine	CGU	(Arg/R) Arginine	U
	CUC		CCC		CAC		CGC		C
	CUA		CCA		CAA	(Gln/Q) Glutamine	CGA		A
	CUG		CCG		CAG		CGG		G
A	AUU	(Ile/I) Isoleucine	ACU	(Thr/T) Threonine	AAU	(Asn/N) Asparagine	AGU	(Ser/S) Serine	U
	AUC		ACC		AAC		AGC		C
	AUA		ACA		AAA	(Lys/K) Lysine	AGA	(Arg/R) Arginine	A
	AUG[A]	(Met/M) Methionine	ACG		AAG		AGG		G
G	GUU	(Val/V) Valine	GCU	(Ala/A) Alanine	GAU	(Asp/D) Aspartic acid	GGU	(Gly/G) Glycine	U
	GUC		GCC		GAC		GGC		C
	GUA		GCA		GAA	(Glu/E) Glutamic acid	GGA		A
	GUG		GCG		GAG		GGG		G

Note that each amino acid is represented by three or more different codons. As a result, even if there is a small mutation in the DNA strand, often there will be no result, because it may end up coding for the same amino acid anyway.

The mRNA is thus read by the ribosome, which receives amino acids carried by t-RNA molecules (transport-RNA). The amino acids are formed into a long polypeptide chain, which after completion, will be folded into a protein.

Step 3: Protein Folding: In the final step, the completed amino acid chain is folded into its correct 3D structure. A protein has 4 types of structure:

- Primary: The primary structure of a protein is the amino acid sequence.
- Secondary: The secondary structure of a protein are the substructures that are formed when protein folding begins. Certain sequences of amino acids are able to form into structures that resemble a sheet, called a beta-sheet, or a helix, called an alpha helix.
- Tertiary: The majority of proteins have a 3D structure called a tertiary structure. This structure is formed from the interaction of all the secondary structures in a protein. Some proteins may be globular, or round in nature, whereas others might be cylindrical or flat.
- Quaternary: Some proteins, but not all, have a quaternary structure. A quaternary structure is one that is an interaction between multiple proteins. For example, the hemoglobin protein, which carries oxygen in blood, will interact as a set of 4 hemoglobin proteins surround iron heme groups.

The proteins which are produced from the DNA transcription and translation process are then exported from the endoplasmic reticulum or freely released into the cytosol, where they can perform their work.

Practice Problems for DNA transcription & Translation

1. Which of the following enzymes is responsible for making a copy of DNA to RNA?
   a) RNA polymerase
   b) DNA polymerase
   c) RNA ligase
   d) DNA helicase

2. If mRNA produced by transcription is used immediately, with no further processing, which of the following would occur?
   a) The protein coded by the mRNA would be functional
   b) The protein coded by the mRNA will not be exported from the cell
   c) The protein coded by the mRNA will not be functional
   d) No polypeptide chain will be produced

3. During transcription, the mRNA is written in which direction?
   a) 5' → 3'
   b) 3' → 5'
   c) 2' → 7'
   d) 7' → 2'

4. When a ribosome reads an mRNA strand, how many base pairs are read at a time?
   a) 1
   b) 2
   c) 3
   d) 4

5. If a single mutation occurs in the third base pair of the codon for histidine, what is the percent chance that the amino acid will be changed?
   a) 0%
   b) 25%
   c) 50%
   d) 66%

Answer Key to Practice Problems

1. A
2. C
3. B
4. C
5. D

Chapter 6: Chemistry

SCIENTIFIC NOTATION

Scientific notation is a method of writing numbers that are either very large, or very small. Traditionally, if we write a large number out in whole, for example: 150,000,000,000, it is very difficult to work with on paper, and also difficult to understand, because we need to count the number of zeroes in order to know how large the number is. Scientific notation offers a shortcut that simplifies a number's written form.

The general format for a scientific notation number is:

$$A \times 10^n$$

"A" is the number in decimal form, and "n" is the "power" of the number. Some examples of common numbers converted to scientific notation are seen in the table below:

Number	Scientific Notation
250	2.5×10^2
1,345,000	1.345×10^6
0.00000458	4.58×10^{-6}
2.5	2.5×10^0

Everything in scientific notation is denoted by a power of 10. In the first example in the table above, we see that 2.5×10^2 is essentially 2.5×100. We want to move the decimal place 2 places to the right to get the full number. For negative powers, we move the decimal place to the left, instead of to the right.

This shortcut is handy for working in chemistry due to the nature of numbers in chemical reactions. For example, one mol of atoms is 6.022×10^{23} atoms. If we were to write out the entire number, we would get:

$$602200000000000000000000$$

This is far too long and confusing for ordinary use. Thus, we use scientific notation. We know that 6.022×10^{23} is 6.022 with the decimal moved 23 places to right (which is a very large number).

When converting a number into scientific notation, the number of significant figures is important, but the size of the number is also import. For example, Avogadro's number's full value is estimated to be:

$$602,214,141,070,409,084,099,072$$

The question here is: which digits are significant? According to the rules of significant figures, nearly all of them should be. However, intuitively, we know that since we are working with such a large number, probably only the first 5 or 6 digits are useful. Any calculation that we do with this number is unlikely to be changed if we include more than the first 5 or 6 digits.

For this reason, when using scientific notation, it is common practice to limit the significant figures to 4. For example, if we were to shorten the number 1,456,892, we would shorten it to 1.456×10^6, not 1.456892×10^6.

Practice Drill: Scientific Notation

1. What is 1.2×10^2 multiplied by 5.5×10^0?
   a) 330
   b) 660
   c) 540
   d) 1020

2. Convert 1,546,250 into scientific notation.
   a) 1.5×10^6
   b) 1.55×10^5
   c) 1.546×10^7
   d) 1.546×10^6

3. What is 0.00545 in scientific notation?
   a) 5.45×10^2
   b) 0.545×10^{-5}
   c) 5.45×10^{-3}
   d) 0.546×10^6

4. When we convert a number to scientific notation, the base number should have a value between:
   a) 0 and 1
   b) 1 and 1.99999 (repeated decimal)
   c) 1 and 9.9999 (repeated decimal)
   d) 1 and 100

5. What is 1 million in scientific notation?
   a) 1×10^3
   b) 1×10^6
   c) 1×10^9
   d) 1×10^{12}

Answer Key to Practice Problems
   1. B
   2. D
   3. C
   4. C
   5. B

METRIC & ENGLISH UNITS

The units of measurement used in calculation are very important to the equations that can be applied, and also to the conversion from one unit size to another. In the scientific community, the metric system of units is the most commonly utilized.

The metric system was developed in the late 1700's, and consists of a prefix + measurement unit. The prefix denotes the "multiplier" or "power" of the number, whereas the measurement unit denotes the property being measured. The below table shows common prefixes and units in the metric system, as well as the counterpart in the English system:

Prefix	Value
Giga	**1,000,000,000**
Mega	**1,000,000**
Kilo	**1,000**
Centi	**0.01**
Milli	**0.001**
Micro	**0.000001**

Metric Unit	English Unit Equivalent	Meaning
Meter	Foot	The meter is the basic measurement unit of **length.**
Gram	Pound	The gram is the basic measurement unit of **mass.**
Joule	BTU (British Thermal Unit)	The joule is the basic measurement unit of **energy.**
Pascal	Atmosphere (atm)	The Pascal is the basic measurement unit of **pressure.**
Celsius	Fahrenheit	The Celsius is the basic measurement unit of **temperature.**

From these two tables, we can look at some examples. The kilojoule, for example, is one thousand (1,000) joules. A kilogram is also 1,000 grams.

It is important to be able to understand the conversion rates between the metric and English units in order to correctly solve problems. These conversion rates can be found online or in most math and science books. Some examples are included below:

1 meter =	3.28 feet
1 kilogram =	2.2 pounds
101,325 Pascals =	1 atmosphere
1055 Joules =	1 Btu
745.7 Watts =	1 horsepower

Finally, one of the most important conversion to understand is the temperature conversion. There are three temperature scales that are used: Celsius, Fahrenheit, and Kelvin.

The Kelvin scale is the "absolute" temperature scale, where 0 K = absolute zero. There is no temperature that exists below 0 Kelvin.

To convert from Kelvin to Celsius, we subtract 273. For example, 273 K = 0 C. 373 K = 100 C, which is the boiling point for water.

To convert Celsius to Fahrenheit, the following calculation can be used:

$$F = 1.8C + 32$$

For example, 15 °C = 59 °F. These conversion are very helpful when performing scientific calculations that involve conversion to different units.

Practice Drill: Metric & English Units

1. If a person weighs 150 lbs, how many kilograms do they weigh?
    a) 75
    b) 65.5
    c) 50.9
    d) 68

2. A student is weighing out some chemicals for an experiment. She weighs out 55 grams of NaCl. How many kilograms is this?
    a) 0.255
    b) 0.55
    c) 0.055
    d) 0.075

3. The average temperature year round in Los Angeles is a sunny 71 degrees Fahrenheit. What is this in Celsius?
    a) 21.7 C
    b) 25.2 C
    c) 11.5 C
    d) 18.1 C

4. If a person is 1.5 meters tall, how many feet tall is he?
    a) 5 feet 11 inches
    b) 4 feet 11 inches
    c) 5 feet 2 inches
    d) 6 feet exactly

5. If you wanted to measure the length of a football field, which of the following units might you use?
    a) Fahrenheit
    b) Joules
    c) Miles
    d) Meters

Answer Key to Practice Problems

1. B
2. C
3. A
4. B
5. D

TEMPERATURE SCALES

There are 4 primary temperature scales that you may come across. They are the Fahrenheit scale, Kelvin scale, Celsius scale, and Rankine scale.

Fahrenheit Scale – The Fahrenheit scale is the standard temperature scale used in the United States. In the Fahrenheit scale, water has a boiling point of 212 °F and a freezing point of 32 °F.

Celsius Scale – The Celsius scale is the standard temperature scale used in the metric system. In the Celsius scale, water has a boiling point of 100 °C and a freezing point of 0 °C.

Kelvin Scale – The Kelvin scale is the secondary temperature scale used in the metric system, and is commonly seen in scientific calculations. Many calculations, such as those for specific heat or those involving the ideal gas constant, use the Kelvin scale. In the Kelvin scale, water has a freezing point of 273 K and a boiling point of 373 K.

Rankine Scale – The Rankine scale is a temperature scale used in the United States, but is not commonly seen anymore. In the Rankine Scale, the freezing point of water is 492 °R and the boiling point is 671 °R.

The below table shows how to convert one temperature scale into another.

	To Fahrenheit	To Celsius	To Kelvin	To Rankine
Fahrenheit	n/a	$[°C]=([°F] - 32) \times \frac{5}{9}$	$[K]=([°F] + 459.67) \times \frac{5}{9}$	$[°R]=[°F] + 459.67$
Celsius	$[°F]=[°C] \times \frac{9}{5} + 32$	n/a	$[K]=[°C] + 273.15$	$[°R]=([°C] + 273.15) \times \frac{9}{5}$
Kelvin	$[°F]=[K] \times \frac{9}{5} - 459.67$	$[°C]=[K] - 273.15$	n/a	$[°R]=[K] \times \frac{9}{5}$
Rankine	$[°F]=[°R] - 459.67$	$[°C]=([°R] - 491.67) \times \frac{5}{9}$	$[K]=[°R] \times \frac{5}{9}$	n/a

Practice Drill: Temperature Scales

1. It's often broiling hot in India during the summer, at a high of 45 °C. What is this temperature in Fahrenheit?
   a) 93
   b) 97
   c) 113
   d) 117

2. Water will commonly have a boiling point of 100 °C, which can be lowered by adding some salt. If the new boiling point is 95 °C, what is this in Kelvin?
   a) 353
   b) 358
   c) 363
   d) 368

3. Which of the following is the hottest temperature?
   a) 235 °R
   b) 95 °C
   c) 389 K
   d) All of these temperatures are the same

4. -20 °C is how much hotter or cooler than -20 °F?
   a) 4 degrees F warmer
   b) 16 degrees F warmer
   c) 4 degrees F cooler
   d) 16 degrees F cooler

5. A student is told to heat her reaction up to 150 °C, but her temperature thermometer is in Rankine! What degree Rankine should the reaction take place at?
   a) 762 R
   b) 568 R
   c) 981 R
   d) 289 R

Answer Key to Practice Problems

1. C
2. D
3. C
4. B
5. A

ELEMENTS, COMPOUNDS, AND MIXTURES

Matter
Matter is commonly defined as anything that takes up space and has mass. **Mass** is the quantity of matter something possesses, and usually has a unit of weight associated with it.

Matter can undergo two types of change: chemical and physical.

> A **chemical change** occurs when an original substance is transformed into a new substance with different properties. An example would be the burning of wood, which produces ash and smoke.

> Transformations that do not produce new substances, such as stretching a rubber band or melting ice, are called **physical changes**.

The fundamental properties which we use to measure matter are mass, weight, volume, density and specific gravity.

Extrinsic properties are directly related to the amount of material being measured, such as weight and volume.

Intrinsic properties are those which are independent of the quantity of matter present, such as density and specific gravity.

Atom
An atom is the ultimate particle of matter; it is the smallest particle of an element that still is a part of that element. All atoms of the same element have the same mass. Atomic chemical changes involve the transfer of whole atoms from one substance to another; but atoms are not created or destroyed in ordinary chemical changes.

An atom is made up of several parts. The center is called the **nucleus**, and is made up of two particles: a positively-charged particle, called a **proton,** and a particle that does not have a charge, called a **neutron**. The masses of a proton and neutron are about the same.

The nucleus of the atom is surrounded by negatively-charged particles called **electrons**, which move in orbits around the nucleus. The nucleus is only a small portion of the total amount of space an atom takes up, even though most of an atom's mass is contained in the nucleus.

Molecular Weight
A **mole** is the amount of substance that contains 6.02×10^{23} basic particles. This is referred to as **Avogadro's number** and is based on the number of atoms in C_{12} (Carbon 12). For example, a mole of copper is the amount of copper that contains exactly 6.02×10^{23} atoms, and one mole of water contains 6.02×10^{23} H_2O molecules. The weight of one mole of an element is called its **atomic weight**. The atomic weight of an element with isotopes, which are explained further below/on the next page[L3], is the average of the isotopes' individual atomic weights.

The negatively-charged electrons are very light in mass. An atom is described as neutral if it has an equal number of protons and electrons, or if the number of electrons is the same as the atomic number of the atom. You may have already assumed – correctly! – from that information that the atomic number of an atom equals the number of protons in that atom. The **atomic weight** or **mass** of the atom is the total number of protons and neutrons in the atom's nucleus.

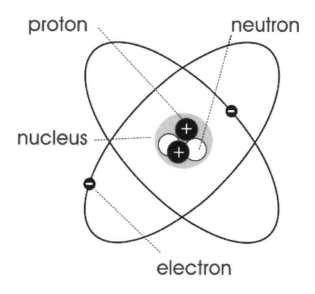

Elements
An element is a substance which cannot be broken down by chemical means; they are composed of atoms that have the same **atomic number** and are defined by the number of protons and neutrons they have. Some elements have more than one form, such as carbon; these alternate forms are called **isotopes.** There are approximately 109 known elements. Eighty-eight of these occur naturally on earth, while the others are **synthesized** (manufactured).

Hydrogen is the most abundant element in the Universe. It is found in 75% of all matter known to exist. **Helium** is the second most abundant element, found in approximately 25% of all known matter. The Earth is composed mostly of iron, oxygen, silicon, and magnesium, though these elements are not evenly distributed. 90% of the human body's mass consists of oxygen, carbon, hydrogen, nitrogen, calcium, and phosphorus. 75% of elements are metals, and eleven are gases in their natural state. We'll cover this more in-depth when we view the periodic table.

Molecules
A molecule is the smallest part of a substance that isn't chemically bonded to another atom. **Chemical formulas** are used to represent the atomic composition of a molecule. For example, one molecule of water contains 2 atoms of Hydrogen and 1 atom of Oxygen; its chemical formula is **$2H + O = H_2O$.**

Compounds and Mixtures
Substances that contain more than one type of element are called **compounds.** Compounds that are made up of molecules which are all identical are called **pure substances.** A **mixture** consists of two or more substances that are not chemically bonded. Mixtures are generally placed in one of two categories:

Homogeneous Mixture: Components that make up the mixture are uniformly distributed; examples are water and air.

Heterogeneous Mixture: Components of the mixture are not uniform; they sometimes have localized regions with different properties. For example: the different components of soup make it a heterogeneous mixture. Rocks, as well, are not uniform and have localized regions with different properties.

A uniform, or homogenous, mixture of different molecules is called a **solution**. If the solution is a liquid, the material being dissolved is the **solute** and the liquid it is being dissolved in is called the **solvent.** Both solids and gases can dissolve in liquids. A **saturated** has reached a point of maximum
concentration; in it, no more solute will dissolve.

Practice Drill: Elements, Compounds, and Mixtures

1. Which statement best describes the density of an atom's nucleus?
   a) The nucleus occupies most of the atom's volume, but contains little of its mass.
   b) The nucleus occupies very little of the atom's volume, and contains little of its mass.
   c) The nucleus occupies most of the atom's volume, and contains most of its mass.
   d) The nucleus occupies very little of the atom's volume, but contains most of its mass.

2. Which of the following is not a physical change?
   a) Melting of aspirin.
   b) Lighting a match.
   c) Putting sugar in tea.
   d) Boiling of antifreeze.

3. A solid melts gradually between 85°C and 95°C to give a milky, oily liquid. When a laser beam shines through the liquid, the path of the beam is clearly visible. The milky liquid is likely to be:
   a) A heterogeneous mixture.
   b) An element.
   c) A compound.
   d) A solution.

4. The identity of an element is determined by:
   a) The number of its protons and neutrons.
   b) The number of its neutrons.
   c) The number of its electrons.
   d) Its atomic mass.

5. True or False? When a match burns, some matter is destroyed.
   a) True.
   b) False.

Practice Drill: Elements, Compounds, and Mixtures – Answers

1. **d)**
2. **b)**
3. **c)**
4. **a)**
5. **b)**

STATES OF MATTER

The physical states of matter are generally grouped into three main categories:

1. **Solids**: Rigid; they maintain their shape and have strong intermolecular forces. Typical solids are rigid at room temperature. In solids, the molecules are closely packed together, and solid materials usually have a high density. In the majority of solids, called crystalline solids, the ions or molecules are packed into a crystal structure that is highly ordered.

2. **Liquids**: Cannot maintain their own shape, conform to their containers, and contain forces strong enough to keep molecules from dispersing into spaces. Solids will generally become liquids when heated to a high enough temperature.

3. **Gases**: Have indefinite shape; disperse rapidly through space due to random movement and are able to occupy any volume. They are held together by weak forces. Gases are produced when liquids are heated enough, and have an additional energy associated with them called the enthalpy of vaporization. This is the energy required to break the liquid bonds, and allow the material to transfer to the gaseous phase.

Two specific states of matter are **liquid crystals**, which can maintain their shape as well as be made to flow, and **plasmas**, gases in which electrons are stripped from their nuclei.

Phase Diagrams

Phase diagrams are used to represent the state of matter depending on the temperature and pressure of the matter. Typically, as temperature drops, a substance is more likely to be a solid, and as pressure drops, a substance is more likely to be a gas. Seen below is an approximate phase diagram for water.

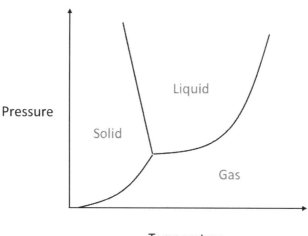

As can be seen, at high pressures and moderate temperatures, gas will be a solid. As temperature increases, water will slowly transition to becoming a liquid, and then a gas. The point at which the three lines meet is called the triple point, which is a state in which the material will exist in all three forms: solid, liquid, and gas. The triple point of water is at 0.01 °C and 0.006 atmospheres of pressure.

Gases

There are four physical properties of gases that are related to each other. If any one of these changes, a change will occur in at least one of the remaining three.

1. Volume of the gas.
2. Pressure of the gas.
3. Temperature of the gas.
4. The number of gas molecules.

The laws that relate these properties to each other are:

Boyle's Law: The volume of a given amount of gas at a constant temperature is inversely proportional to pressure. In other words; if the initial volume decreases by half, the pressure will double and vice versa. The representative equation is: $P_1V_1 = P_2V_2$.

Charles's Law: The volume of a given amount of gas at a constant pressure is directly proportional to absolute (Kelvin) temperature. If the temperature of the gas increases, the volume of the gas also increases and vice versa. The representative equation is: $V_1/T_1 = V_2/T_2$.

Avogadro's Law: Equal volumes of all gases under identical conditions of pressure and temperature contain the same number of molecules. The molar volume of all ideal gases at 0° C and a pressure of 1 atm. is 22.4 liters.

The **kinetic theory of gases** assumes that gas molecules are very small compared to the distance between the molecules. Gas molecules are in constant, random motion; they frequently collide with each other and with the walls of whatever container they are in.

Ideal Gas Law

The ideal gas law is an important equation that is used to estimate the properties of gas at different temperatures and pressures. It is called the ideal gas law because in order for it to be effective, the gas must be ideal, meaning that:

1. The gas consists of a large number of molecules that move randomly.
2. The volume that the molecules of the gas occupies is very small compared to the total volume of the gas.
3. There are no attractive or repulsive interactions between the gas molecules.

The Ideal Gas Law can be stated as:

$$PV = nRT$$

Where P is the pressure, V is the volume, n is the number of mols of gas, R is the ideal gas constant (8.314 J/mol K) and T is the temperature.

Practice Drill: States of Matter

1. Under the same conditions of pressure and temperature, a liquid differs from a gas because the molecules of the liquid:
    a) Have no regular arrangement.
    b) Are in constant motion.
    c) Have stronger forces of attraction between them.
    d) Take the shape of the container they are in.

2. Methane (CH_4) gas diffuses through air because the molecules are:
    a) Moving randomly.
    b) Dissolving quickly.
    c) Traveling slowly.
    d) Expanding steadily.

3. Which of the following would not change if the number of gas molecules changed?
    a) Volume of the gas.
    b) Type of gas.
    c) Pressure of the gas.
    d) Temperature of gas.

4. When the pressure is increased on a can filled with gas, its volume _____.
    a) Stays the same.
    b) Increases.
    c) Decreases.
    d) Turns to liquid.

5. Equal volumes of all gases at the same temperature and pressure contain the same number of molecules. This statement is known as:
    a) Kinetic theory of gases.
    b) Charles's Law.
    c) Boyle's Law.
    d) Avogadro's Law.

Practice Drill: States of Matter – Answers

1. **c)**
2. **a)**
3. **b)**
4. **c)**
5. **d)**

ATOMIC MASS & STRUCTURE

An atom is composed of three individual units: protons, neutrons and electrons.

Proton – A proton is a particle with one atomic mass unit, which is roughly equivalent to $1.660538921 \times 10^{-27}$ kg. It possesses a +1 positive charge, and is one of the key determinants in the properties of an element. Elements are arranged in order of their number of protons, starting with hydrogen, which has only 1 proton. The atomic number of an element is related to the number of protons it has. For example, iron, which has an atomic number of 26, has exactly 26 protons.

Neutron – A neutron is a particle which also has one atomic mass unit, but is not charged (hence its name, derived from 'neutral'). The neutron content in an element is variable. For example, the majority of carbon atoms have 6 neutrons, but some of them have 7 neutrons. The additional neutron gives carbon-13 some radioactive properties. The added radioactivity is also seen in many elements which have more neutrons that normal.

Electron – An electron is a particle which has a -1 charge, and a mass much smaller than that of a proton, estimated to be about $9.10938291 \times 10^{-31}$ kg. Electrons do not make up much of the mass of an atom. Electrons are contained within the electron shell of an atom, and are constantly in movement.

Combined, these three units make up an atom. We can understand the composition of these three units by looking at information given in a periodic table. Let's look at oxygen below in the periodic table:

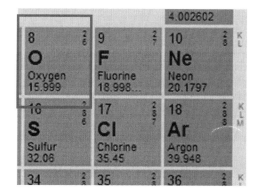

- The number in the upper left is the atomic number: 8. This means oxygen has 8 protons.
- The number in the lower left is the atomic mass: 15.999. this means oxygen weighs 16 atomic mass units.
- The number in the upper right is the number of electrons in its S-shell: 2
- The number below that is the number of electrons in its total valence shell: 6. This means, for example, that oxygen needs 2 more electrons to fill its valence shell of 8.

In order to find out how many neutrons an element has, subtract its atomic mass from its atomic number. In the case of oxygen, we see that 16-8 = 8 neutrons.

Practice Drill: Atomic Mass & Structure

1. How many electrons are in the valence shell of sulfur?
   a) 2
   b) 4
   c) 6
   d) 8

2. How many neutrons does the element Molybdenum have?
   a) 26
   b) 27
   c) 54
   d) 55

3. An isotope of nitrogen has 8 neutrons instead of 7. What is the weight of 1 mol of this isotope?
   a) 13 grams
   b) 14 grams
   c) 15 grams
   d) 16 grams

4. Approximately how many times more massive is a proton compared to an electron?
   a) About 1000 times
   b) About 2000 times
   c) About 4000 times
   d) About 8000 times

5. What is the number of protons, neutrons, and electrons, respectively, in a silicon atom?
   a) 14, 14, 8
   b) 12, 12, 14
   c) 14, 12, 8
   d) 14, 14, 14

Answer Key to Practice Problems

   1. C
   2. C
   3. C
   4. B
   5. D

PERIODIC TABLE AND CHEMICAL BONDS

The Periodic table

The Periodic Table is a chart which arranges the chemical elements in a useful, logical manner. Elements are listed in order of increasing atomic number, lined up so that elements which exhibit similar properties are arranged in the same row or column as each other.

hydrogen 1 **H** 1.0079																	helium 2 **He** 4.0026
lithium 3 **Li** 6.941	beryllium 4 **Be** 9.0122											boron 5 **B** 10.811	carbon 6 **C** 12.011	nitrogen 7 **N** 14.007	oxygen 8 **O** 15.999	fluorine 9 **F** 18.998	neon 10 **Ne** 20.180
sodium 11 **Na** 22.990	magnesium 12 **Mg** 24.305											aluminium 13 **Al** 26.982	silicon 14 **Si** 28.086	phosphorus 15 **P** 30.974	sulfur 16 **S** 32.065	chlorine 17 **Cl** 35.453	argon 18 **Ar** 39.948
potassium 19 **K** 39.098	calcium 20 **Ca** 40.078	scandium 21 **Sc** 44.956	titanium 22 **Ti** 47.867	vanadium 23 **V** 50.942	chromium 24 **Cr** 51.996	manganese 25 **Mn** 54.938	iron 26 **Fe** 55.845	cobalt 27 **Co** 58.933	nickel 28 **Ni** 58.693	copper 29 **Cu** 63.546	zinc 30 **Zn** 65.39	gallium 31 **Ga** 69.723	germanium 32 **Ge** 72.61	arsenic 33 **As** 74.922	selenium 34 **Se** 78.96	bromine 35 **Br** 79.904	krypton 36 **Kr** 83.80
rubidium 37 **Rb** 85.468	strontium 38 **Sr** 87.62	yttrium 39 **Y** 88.906	zirconium 40 **Zr** 91.224	niobium 41 **Nb** 92.906	molybdenum 42 **Mo** 95.94	technetium 43 **Tc** [98]	ruthenium 44 **Ru** 101.07	rhodium 45 **Rh** 102.91	palladium 46 **Pd** 106.42	silver 47 **Ag** 107.87	cadmium 48 **Cd** 112.41	indium 49 **In** 114.82	tin 50 **Sn** 118.71	antimony 51 **Sb** 121.76	tellurium 52 **Te** 127.60	iodine 53 **I** 126.90	xenon 54 **Xe** 131.29
caesium 55 **Cs** 132.91	barium 56 **Ba** 137.33	57-70 ✱	lutetium 71 **Lu** 174.97	hafnium 72 **Hf** 178.49	tantalum 73 **Ta** 180.95	tungsten 74 **W** 183.84	rhenium 75 **Re** 186.21	osmium 76 **Os** 190.23	iridium 77 **Ir** 192.22	platinum 78 **Pt** 195.08	gold 79 **Au** 196.97	mercury 80 **Hg** 200.59	thallium 81 **Tl** 204.38	lead 82 **Pb** 207.2	bismuth 83 **Bi** 208.98	polonium 84 **Po** [209]	astatine 85 **At** [210]	radon 86 **Rn** [222]
francium 87 **Fr** [223]	radium 88 **Ra** [226]	89-102 ✱✱	lawrencium 103 **Lr** [262]	rutherfordium 104 **Rf** [261]	dubnium 105 **Db** [262]	seaborgium 106 **Sg** [266]	bohrium 107 **Bh** [264]	hassium 108 **Hs** [269]	meitnerium 109 **Mt** [268]	ununnilium 110 **Uun** [271]	unununium 111 **Uuu** [272]	ununbium 112 **Uub** [277]		ununquadium 114 **Uuq** [289]			

✱ Lanthanide series

lanthanum 57 **La** 138.91	cerium 58 **Ce** 140.12	praseodymium 59 **Pr** 140.91	neodymium 60 **Nd** 144.24	promethium 61 **Pm** [145]	samarium 62 **Sm** 150.36	europium 63 **Eu** 151.96	gadolinium 64 **Gd** 157.25	terbium 65 **Tb** 158.93	dysprosium 66 **Dy** 162.50	holmium 67 **Ho** 164.93	erbium 68 **Er** 167.26	thulium 69 **Tm** 168.93	ytterbium 70 **Yb** 173.04

✱✱ Actinide series

actinium 89 **Ac** [227]	thorium 90 **Th** 232.04	protactinium 91 **Pa** 231.04	uranium 92 **U** 238.03	neptunium 93 **Np** [237]	plutonium 94 **Pu** [244]	americium 95 **Am** [243]	curium 96 **Cm** [247]	berkelium 97 **Bk** [247]	californium 98 **Cf** [251]	einsteinium 99 **Es** [252]	fermium 100 **Fm** [257]	mendelevium 101 **Md** [258]	nobelium 102 **No** [259]

Note the following characteristics:

Each box contains the symbol of the element, its atomic number, and its atomic weight.

The elements appear in increasing order according to their atomic numbers, except for the two separate rows.

The vertical columns are called **groups**. Elements within a group share several common properties and often have the same outer electron arrangement. There are two categories: the main group and the transition elements.

> The number of the main group corresponds to the number of valence electrons. Most of the transition elements contain 2 electrons in their valence shells.

The horizontal rows are called **periods** and correspond to the number of occupied electron shells of the atom.

The elements set below the main table are the **lanthanoids** (upper row) and **actinoids**. They also usually have two electrons in their outer shells.

Most of the elements on the periodic table are metals. The alkali metals, alkaline earths, basic metals, transition metals, lanthanides, and actinides are all groups of metals.

In general, the elements increase in mass from left to right and from top to bottom.

The main difference between the modern periodic table and the one Mendeleev (the periodic table's creator) came up with is that Mendeleev's original table arranged the elements in order of increasing atomic weight, while the modern table orders the elements by increasing atomic number.

Electronic Structure of Atoms

The electrons of an atom have fixed energy levels. Those in the principle energy levels are said to be in **electron shells**. Shells which correspond to the highest energy levels, called **valence shells**, include the electrons usually involved in chemical bonding. Chemical formulas of simple compounds can often be predicted from valences. The valence electrons increase in number as you go across the periodic table.

The electrons in the outer orbit can combine with other atoms by giving up electrons or taking on electrons. Atoms that give up electrons (**cations**) change from being neutral to having a *positive* charge. Atoms that gain electrons (**ions**) change from being neutral to having a *negative* charge. The **octet rule** is a chemical rule which states that atoms of a low atomic number will share, gain, or lose electrons in order to fill outer electron shells with eight electrons. This is achieved through different types of bonding.

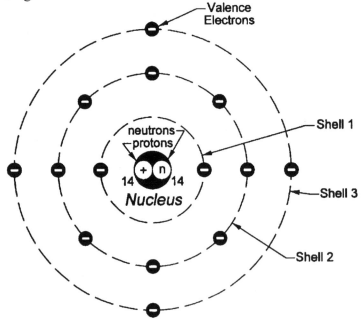

Chemical Bonds

Electromagnetism is involved in all chemical behavior, including the chemical bonds which hold atoms together to form molecules, as well as those holding molecules together to form all substances. **Electronegativity** measures the tendency of an atom to attract a bonding pair of electrons, and is affected by both the atomic number, and the distance between the valence electrons and the charged nucleus. The higher the assigned electronegativity number, the more an element or compound attracts electrons.

There are two main types of bonds formed between atoms: **Ionic** and **Covalent bonds.** Anions and cations, being negatively and positively charged respectively, exist because of the attraction of opposite charges, and usually form **ionic bonds**.

A covalent bond forms when atoms share valence electrons. However, atoms do not always share electrons equally, resulting in a **polar covalent bond**. Electrons shared by two metallic atoms, form a **metallic bond**. Those electrons participating in metallic bonds may be shared between any of the metal atoms in the region.

If the electronegativity values of two atoms are similar, then:
- Metallic bonds form between two metal atoms.
- Covalent bonds form between two non-metal atoms.
- Non-polar covalent bonds form when the electronegativity values are very similar.
- Polar covalent bonds form when the electronegativity values are a little further apart.

If the electronegativity values of two atoms are different, then ionic bonds are formed.

Most metals have less than 4 valence electrons, which allows them to either gain a few electrons or lose a few; they generally tend to lose electrons, which causes them to become more positive. (This means that metals tend to form cations.)

A **hydrogen bond** is not considered a chemical bond. Instead, in a hydrogen bond, the attractive force between hydrogen is attached to an electronegative atom of one molecule and an electronegative atom of a different molecule. Usually the electronegative atom is oxygen, nitrogen, or fluorine, which have partial negative charges. The hydrogen has the partial positive charge. Hydrogen bonds are much weaker than both ionic and covalent bonds.

Multiple Bonding Patterns

Depending on the electron structure of the atom, double or even triple bonds are possible between atoms. Double and triple bonds share 4 and 6 electrons between a pair of atoms, respectively. These types of bonds are usually quite stable. For example, O_2 possesses a double bond and N_2 possesses a triple bond. An example of a larger molecule with a double or triple bond is seen below:

$(CH_3)_2C=CHCH_2C(CH_3)_3$

2,5,5-trimethyl-2-hexene

The double bond structure is represented in chemistry by a pair of parallel lines, rather than the single line seen for a normal bond. In the molecule above, the double bond is located between the 2nd and 3rd carbon in the hexane molecule.

VSEPR Bonding Theory

VSEPR, short for Valence Shell Electron Pair Repulsion theory is a method that aids in understanding the three dimensional structure of a molecule. According to the repulsion of each pair of electrons in a bond, we can understand how a molecule's geometry will look like. The basic forms of geometry are:

- **Linear** – When there are 3 atoms in a molecule that have no high electronegativity differences, the molecule is linear:

X——A——X

- **Trigonal Planar** – Seen in molecules with four atoms that may have a lone pair on each end:

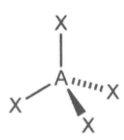

- **Tetrahedral** – The tetrahedral molecule is the standard shape for a single central atom surround by 4 bonds. The bond angles between the different atoms may be different due to electronegativity differences.

X
|
A
X⟋ ⟍X
X

There are additional bonding structures, such as trigonal bipyrimidal (6 total atoms), octahedral, and pentagonal. However, these bonding structures are not common in day to day chemical reactions.

Practice Drill: Periodic Table and Chemical Bonds

1. When cations and anions join, they form what kind of chemical bond?
   a) Ionic.
   b) Hydrogen.
   c) Metallic.
   d) Covalent.

2. Generally, how do atomic masses vary throughout the periodic table of the elements?
   a) They decrease from left to right and increase from top to bottom.
   b) They increase from left to right and increase bottom to top.
   c) They increase from left to right and increase top to bottom.
   d) They increase from right to left and decrease bottom to top.

3. The force involved in all chemical behavior is:
   a) Electronegativity.
   b) Covalent bonds.
   c) Electromagnetism.
   d) Ionic bonds.

4. Which one of the following is not a form of chemical bonding?
   a) Covalent bonding.
   b) Hydrogen bonding.
   c) Ionic bonding.
   d) Metallic bonding.

5. Two atoms which do not share electrons equally will form what type of bond?
   a) Metallic bonds.
   b) Polar covalent.
   c) Ionic bonds.
   d) They cannot form bonds.

6. Chemical bonding:
   a) Uses electrons that are closest to the nucleus of the atoms bonding.
   b) Always uses electrons from only one of the atoms involved.
   c) Uses all the electrons in all atoms involved.
   d) Uses the valence electrons of all the atoms involved.

Practice Drill: Periodic Table and Chemical Bonds – Answers

1. a)
2. c)
3. c)
4. b)
5. b)
6. d)

CHANGES IN STATE: VAPORIZATION/CONDENSATION

A material can change from one state, such as liquid, to another state, such as gas, depending on the surrounding temperature and pressure. In most conditions that we see, the pressure is atmospheric, and as a general rule, as temperature increases, the state will progress from solid to liquid to gas, and the opposite will occur as temperature decreases.

Terminology to know:

Boiling point: The boiling point is also the point of vaporization of a material. For example, the boiling point of water is 100 °C at normal atmospheric pressure. Thus, at 100 °C liquid water will turn into water vapor.

Freezing point: The freezing point is also the melting point of a solid. For example, the melting/freezing point of water is 0 °C.

Critical point: The critical point is the temperature and pressure at which defined states do not exist. For example, at the critical point of water, which happens at 374°C and 218 atmospheres, there is no defined state for water. It is considered "plasma", and behaves with different properties than either liquid or gas.

Latent heat: The latent heat of vaporization is the heat required for a liquid to turn into a gas. Below is a table showing example values of latent heat for some common substances.

Substance	Latent heat of Vaporization	Boiling Point (C)
Ethanol	855 kJ/kg	78.3
Water	2260 kJ/kg	100
Nitrogen	200 kJ/kg	-196

In these examples provided, we can understand the following:

The energy that is in 1 kilogram of water vapor is 2,260 kJ more than in 1 kilogram of liquid water.

Specific Heat

The specific heat of a substance is the amount of energy it requires to raise the substance by 1 unit of temperature. For example, the specific heat of water is about 4.19 J/g*K. This means that you need 4.19 Joules of energy to heat 1 gram of water by 1 degree centigrade. The specific heat is a useful property that can be used to predict the amount of energy needed to heat up a substance. For example, if you want to warm a 100 mL (100 g) cup of water from 25 °C to 50 °C, you would need about 10,450 joules of energy.

Practice Drill – Changes in State

1. What is the correct term for the energy required for a solid to become a liquid?
   a) Latent heat of vaporization
   b) Latent heat of fusion
   c) Latent heat of fission
   d) None of the above

2. A student wishes to boil 0.5 kg of water, about half a liter. After the water reaches 100 °C, how much more energy is required for it to boil?
   a) 760 kJ
   b) 960 kJ
   c) 1130 kJ
   d) 2240 kJ

3. Which of the following is not a state of matter?
   a) Plasma
   b) Liquid
   c) Solid
   d) All of the above are states of matter

4. A student has a cup of water at room temperature 25 °C and 1 atm. He notices the temperature in the room is rapidly increasing! How might he keep the water in liquid state and prevent it from vaporizing?
   a) Further increasing the temperature
   b) Increasing the pressure in the room
   c) Decreasing the pressure in the room
   d) Mixing the water very quickly

5. What is the best definition of a solution?
   a) A mixture of a solute dissolved in a solvent
   b) A combination of more than 3 elements in a liquid form
   c) Any pure, liquid, element
   d) None of the above can be classified as a solution

6. Which of the following is the process that produces a liquid from a gas?
   a) Vaporization
   b) Condensation
   c) Sublimation
   d) Denitrification

Answer Key to Practice Drill
   1. B
   2. C
   3. D
   4. B
   5. A
   6. B

149

CHEMICAL REACTIONS

A chemical reaction occurs when there is a conversion of one set of chemical substances to another set. Chemical reactions are caused primarily by a change in bonding structure in these substances due to the exchange of electrons.

In a chemical reaction, the starting substances are called the reagents, and the ending substances are called the products. In the reaction below, sodium hydroxide reacts with iron sulfate to form sodium sulfate and iron hydroxide, the products.

$$2NaOH + FeSO_4 \rightarrow Na_2SO_4 + Fe(OH)_2$$

The above reaction is known as a double displacement reaction. In double displacement reactions, there are two reagents which interact to form two products. The ions from *both* reagents are displaced, hence the name double displacement. There are also 5 other primary types of chemical reactions:

1. Combustion reaction – A combustion reaction occurs when oxygen is reacted in the presence of heat to a combustible compound, usually an organic compound. The products of a combustion reaction are always water and carbon dioxide. For example, the reaction of methane with oxygen will proceed as follows:

$$CH_4 + 2\,O_2 \rightarrow CO_2 + 2H_2O$$

2. Synthesis reaction – This is the most simple reaction in the book. Two compounds, usually elements, combine to form a third compound, the product:

$$C + O_2 \rightarrow CO_2$$

3. Decomposition reaction – This is the opposite of a synthesis reaction, and is usually endothermic. In the decomposition reaction, a single compound decomposes to form two new compounds.

4. Single Displacement reaction – Similar to the double displacement reaction seen above, but only one reactive species changes. For example:

$$MgCl_2 + 2Na \rightarrow Mg + 2NaCl$$

5. Acid Base reaction – In an acid base reaction, one of two reactive species must be seen: a hydrogen ion (H+), or a hydroxide ion (OH-). Hydrogen ions are acidic in nature, and hydroxide ions are basic in nature. When combined, the two ions react to form water.

Energy States

Chemical reactions are influenced by the energy state of the reagents and the products, and a chemical reaction is much more likely to occur if the energy state of the products is *lower* than the energy state of the reactants. However, even if the energy state of the products is higher than that of the reactants, energy can be put into the chemical reaction in order to force it to occur. This highlights two primary types of reactions:

Endothermic reaction: Chemical reactions can be endothermic, meaning heat absorbing. An endothermic reaction requires an input of energy before the reaction can start. A majority of chemical reactions are endothermic. For example, although air will react with metal to form rust, the reaction is endothermic in nature, and will occur either slowly or not at all. This is why your table and chair don't fall apart in the air.

Exothermic reaction: A chemical reaction that is exothermic, or heat releasing, will release energy during its course, forming lower energy products. These reactions are spontaneous, and do not require added energy.

Reaction Stoichiometry

Stoichiometry is the ratio of different compounds taking part in a reaction. The reaction stoichiometry is the relative ratio of each of the reactants and products in a reaction. Stoichiometry is used to determine the amount of products that can be formed from a given set of reactants.

For example, in the single displacement reaction shown above:

$$MgCl_2 + 2Na \rightarrow Mg + 2NaCl$$

1 mol of magnesium chloride in addition to 2 mols of sodium are required in the reactants. This then creates 1 mol of magnesium and 2 mols of sodium chloride.

Reaction stoichiometry can be used to predict the amount of products formed. Given the reaction:

$$C_2H_8 + 4O_2 \rightarrow ?$$

This is a combustion reaction. How many mols of carbon dioxide and water are formed?

To answer this question, we can follow these steps:
1. Convert masses to mols (In this case, we already have mol values, so this is not necessary. In some problems, however, mass values will be given)
2. Write and balance the equation:

We know that this is a combustion reaction, so the reaction should be:

$$C_2H_8 + 4O_2 \rightarrow CO_2 + H_2O$$

However, this is not balanced. There are more atoms on the left than the right. We see that we need to have 2 carbon dioxide molecules and 4 water molecules in order for the mass balance to be correct. This gives us:

$$C_2H_8 + 4O_2 \rightarrow 2CO_2 + 4H_2O$$

We can check and see that the reaction stoichiometry is correct. There are the same number of carbons, hydrogens, and oxygen on the left as there are on the right.

3. Convert mols back to mass if necessary.

Practice Drill – Chemical Reactions

1. In your home, natural gas (methane) is burned to produce heat to keep the house warm. What sort of reaction is this?
    a) Acid base reaction
    b) Combustion reaction
    c) Single displacement reaction
    d) Synthesis reaction

2. A student mixes two unknown chemicals into a beaker (don't do this at home!). He notices that the beaker gets really hot. What type of reaction is this?
    a) Exothermic
    b) Endothermic
    c) Combustion
    d) Reaction

3. Which of the following is a substance or compound that is entering into a reaction?
    a) Mol
    b) Reactant
    c) Product
    d) Chemical

4. Acid rain is produced from the interaction of water and sulfur trioxide. Sulfur trioxide (SO_3) is produced when sulfur is burned. Which of the following is the correct general reaction for this process?
    a) Sulfur + nitrogen → sulfur trioxide
    b) Sulfur + oxygen → sulfur dioxide
    c) Sulfur dioxide + oxygen → sulfur trioxide
    d) Sulfur + oxygen → sulfur trioxide

5. In a balanced equation:
    a) The mass of the reactants equals the mass of the products
    b) The number of mols of reactants equals the number of mols of the products
    c) The size of each molecule in the reaction remains the same
    d) None of the above are correct

6. What type of reaction is the following?

$$CaCl_2 + 2NaOH \rightarrow Ca(OH)_2 + 2NaCl$$

a) Single replacement
b) Double replacement
c) Synthesis
d) Acid Base

Answer Key to Practice Drill

1. B
2. A
3. B
4. D
5. A
6. B

OXIDATION & REDUCTION REACTIONS

Oxidation/reduction reactions (also known as redox reactions) are chemical reactions that result in atoms or molecules having their oxidation state changed.

The oxidation state of an atom is the degree of oxidation in an atom. A positive oxidation state indicates that an atom does not have enough electrons to maintain a neutral condition. For example, the atom Fe^{2+} is missing 2 electrons. A negative oxidation state indicates that an atom has too many electrons. For example, Cl^- has one extra electron, giving it a negative charge.

An increase in the oxidation state (loss of electrons) is known as an oxidation reaction.

A decrease in the oxidation state (gain of electrons) is known as a reduction reaction.

In an oxidation/reduction reaction, one or more reactive species is oxidized, and one or more reactive species is reduced. A helpful mnemonic to remember how redox reactions can be classified is OIL RIG, as seen below:

Oxidation Involves Loss, Reduction Involves Gain

Note that this terminology is focused on the reactants themselves. Conversely, a reactant that takes electrons from another reactant is known as an oxidizer. Good oxidizers include highly electronegative elements, or molecules with a high oxidation state. A reactant that gives away electrons is being oxidized, but the reactant itself is a reducer.

Species – Gives away electrons = reducer, and is being oxidized
Species – Takes electrons = oxidizer, and is being reduced

A simple example of an oxidation/reduction reaction is worked out below:

$$H_2 + F_2 \rightarrow 2HF$$
Which species is being oxidized, and which is being reduced?

First, we assess the individual atoms. Hydrogen has only one valence electron and is likely to lose it, becoming oxidized. Fluorine has 7 valence electrons, and wants to gain one more for a full shell, and is likely to become reduced.

Half reactions written out:

$$H_2 \rightarrow 2H^+ + 2e^-$$
$$F_2 + 2e^- \rightarrow 2F^-$$

$$H_2 + F_2 \rightarrow 2H^+ + 2F^- \rightarrow 2HF$$

From the written out reactions, we can clearly see that fluorine is gaining an electron and being reduced, and hydrogen is losing an electron, and is being oxidized.

Sometimes, the elements or molecules in a compound already have an oxidation state. The best way to determine this oxidation state is according to the electronegativity and the valence shell tendency, as described above. For example:

What is the oxidation state of calcium in the compound $CaSO_4$?

We recognize that calcium has 2 electrons in its valence shell, and is likely to give them up. Additionally, the charge on the SO_4 group is usually -2. Thus, we can state that calcium's oxidative state is +2.

Additionally, we can ask: what is the oxidation state of sulfur in this compound?

We know that oxygen normally has a oxidation state of -2, and we know that calcium has an oxidation state of +2.

Looking at this, we can see that:

$Ca^{2+} + 3O^{2-}$ gives us a total oxidation state of -4. Since we know that $CaSO_4$ is not charged, we conclude that sulfur has an oxidation state of +4 in this compound.

Practice Drill – Redox Reactions

1. Consider the compound NH_4Cl. What is the oxidation state of the nitrogen atom?
   a) -1
   b) -2
   c) -3
   d) -4

2. What is the oxidation state of iron formed in rust, Fe_2O_3?
   a) +2
   b) +3
   c) +4
   d) +6

3. Which of the following compounds is *not* likely to be an oxidizer?
   a) O_2
   b) HCl
   c) Mg
   d) Cl_2

4. In the following reaction, which species is being reduced?

   $Zn + 2HCl \rightarrow ZnCl_2 + H_2$

   a) Zinc
   b) Chlorine
   c) Hydrogen
   d) None of the species has been reduced

5. One of the following statements regarding oxidation/reduction reactions is *not* true. Which is it?
   a) A reduction reaction must occur if an oxidation reaction has occurred.
   b) Compounds which have a positive oxidation state will usually bond to those with a negative oxidation state.
   c) In redox reactions, a transfer of electrons must occur.
   d) Only elements missing 1 or 2 electrons can participate in redox reactions.

6. In the following reaction, what is the correct half reaction for the magnesium oxide species?

   $MnO_2 + 4HCl \rightarrow Cl_2 + 2H_2O + MnCl_2$

   a) $MnO_2 + 2e^- \rightarrow Mn^{2+} + 2O^{2-}$
   b) $MnO_2 \rightarrow Mn^{2+} + 2O^{2-} + 2e^-$
   c) $MnO_2 + 2e^- \rightarrow Mn + 2O$
   d) $MnO_2 + 2e^- \rightarrow Mn^{2-} + 2O^{2+}$

Answer Key for Practice Drill

1. C
2. B
3. C
4. C
5. D
6. A

ACIDS AND BASES

Acids

Naturally-occurring **acid solutions**, in which the solvent is always water, have several characteristic properties in common. They have a sour taste; speed up the corrosion, or rusting, of metals; conduct electricity; and introduce H^+ cations into aqueous solutions.

These characteristic properties can be changed by the addition of a base.

Bases (Alkalis)

Bases don't occur in as many common materials as do acids. A few examples of bases are: lime, lye, and soap. Basic solutions, as opposed to acidic solutions, have a bitter taste; conduct electricity, when their solvent is water; and introduce OH^- ions into an aqueous solution.

The characteristic properties can be changed by the addition of an acid.

The acidity or basicity of a solution is expressed by **pH values**. A neutral solution is defined by the following: it has equal concentrations of H^+ cations and OH^- ions, and a pH of 7. Neutrality is based on the pH of pure water. The more acidic a solution, the lower the pH is below 7. The more basic the solution, the higher the pH is above 7. The pH scale is based on logarithms of base 10. (If one solution has a pH of 8 and another has a pH of 10, then there is a 10^2 or 100 fold difference between the two.)

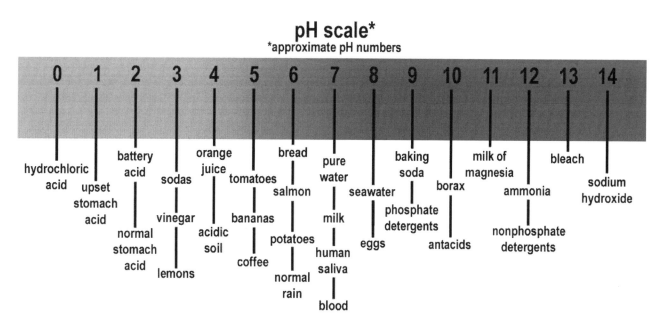

A **buffer** is used to make a solution which exhibits very little change in its pH when small amounts of an acid or base are added to it.

An acidic buffer solution is simply one which has a pH less than 7. Acidic buffer solutions are commonly made from a weak acid and one of its salts - often a sodium salt. A strong basic solution can be weakened by adding an acidic buffer.

An alkaline buffer solution has a pH greater than 7. Alkaline buffer solutions are commonly made from a weak base and one of its salts. A strong acid can be made weaker by adding an alkaline buffer.

The human body contains many enzymes that only function at a specific pH. Once outside of this range, the enzymes are either unable to catalyze reactions or, in some cases, will break down. Our bodies produce a buffer solution that is a mixture of carbonic acid and bicarbonate, in order to keep the pH of blood at 7.4.

Practice Drill: Acids and Bases

1. One of the characteristic properties of an acid is that they introduce:
   a) Hydrogen ions.
   b) Hydroxyl ions.
   c) Hydride ions.
   d) Oxide ions.

2. A solution with a pH of 12 is:
   a) Very acidic.
   b) Neutral.
   c) Very basic.
   d) You can't have a solution with a pH of 12.

3. Buffers keep the pH of a solution from changing by:
   a) Converting strong acids to weak ones.
   b) Converting weak acids to strong ones.
   c) Converting weak bases to strong ones.
   d) More than one of the above answers is correct.

4. Proper blood pH level for humans is:
   a) 7.0.
   b) 7.2.
   c) 7.6.
   d) 7.4.

5. All of the following are properties of alkalis except:
   a) Bitter taste.
   b) Basic solutions are high conductors of electricity.
   c) Introduce OH⁻ ions into an aqueous solution.
   d) The characteristic properties can be changed by the addition of an acid.

Practice Drill: Acids and Bases – Answers

1. **a)**
2. **c)**
3. **a)**
4. **d)**
5. **b)**

Chapter 7: Anatomy & Physiology

Anatomy and Physiology are the studies of body parts and body systems. This section will cover all necessary medical terms, word parts and terminology, as well as the anatomy and physiology of each body system.

Structure Hierarchy of the Human Body

- Organsim
    - Organ Systems
        - Organs
            - Tissues
                - Cells
                    - Molecules
                        - Atoms

Directional Terms

Superior	Toward the head, or toward the upper body region
Inferior	Toward the lower body region
Anterior (Ventral)	On the belly or front side of the body
Posterior (Dorsal)	On the buttocks or back side of the body
Proximal	Near the trunk or middle part of the body
Distal	Furthest away from the point of reference
Medial	Close to the midline of the body
Lateral	Away from the midline of the body

Word Parts
A medical term often has three parts: the prefix, the root, and suffix.

- Prefix - Begins the word, modifies the root, and not a part of all medical terms.
  Example: hyperactive; hyper- modifies the word active.

- Root - Center part of the word, holds meaning, and is often referred to as the "body" of the word.
  Example: Tonsillectomy; tonsil is the root word.

- Suffix - Ends the word, modifies the root, refers to a procedure, action, or condition, and is not part of all medical terms.
  Example: Vasectomy; -ectomy modifies the root word vas.

Prefixes

epi-	on/upon
hyper-	over
hypo-	under
intra-	within
para-	beside
per-	through
peri-	surrounding
sub-	under

Suffixes

-coccus	spherical bacterium
-ia	condition
-ectomy	removal
-malacia	softening
-tome	an instrument to cut
-tomy	to cut
-rrhea	discharge
-plasty	surgical repair
-opsy	view of

Body Cavities

- Cranial cavity - Contains the brain
- Spinal cavity - Contains the spinal cord, and extends from the brainstem in the cranial cavity to the end of the spinal cord
- Thoracic cavity - Contains the lungs, heart, and large blood vessels, and is separated from the abdomen by the diaphragm
- Abdominal cavity - Contains the stomach, intestines, liver, gallbladder, pancreas, spleen, and kidneys, and is separated from the thoracic cavity by the diaphragm
- Pelvic cavity - Contains the urinary bladder, urinary structures, and reproductive organs

The Circulatory System

The circulatory system is vital to human functioning. It is composed of the cardiovascular and pulmonary systems. The cardiovascular system includes the heart, blood, and blood vessels. This is where circulation begins, ends, and begins again. The pulmonary system is composed of the lungs and muscles that allow breathing.

The cardiovascular system plays a vital role in the functioning of humans, as it distributes oxygen, nutrients and hormones to the entire body. The whole system relies on the heart, a muscular organ that is no bigger than a closed fist. The heart must pump the blood low in oxygen to the lungs, and once the blood is in the lungs, it is oxygenated and returned to the heart. The heart then pumps the oxygenated blood through the whole body.

A. The Heart

The *heart* is the muscular organ located inside the rib cage. It can be found approximately between the second and the sixth rib from the bottom of the rib cage. The heart does not sit on the body's midline. Rather, two-thirds of it is located on the left side of the body. Other facts about the heart include:

- It is slightly cone shaped.

- The narrower part of the heart is called the *apex,* and it points downwards and to the left of the body.

- The broader part of the heart is called the *base,* and it points upwards.

The cavity that holds the heart is called the pericardial cavity. It is filled with serous fluid produced by the pericardium, which is the lining of the pericardial cavity. The serous fluid acts as a lubricant for the heart. It also keeps the heart in place and empties the space around the heart.

1. Three Layers of the Heart Wall

- *Epicardium* – This is the outermost layer of the heart, and is one of the two layers of the pericardium.

- *Myocardium* – This is the middle layer of the heart that contains the cardiac muscular tissue. It performs the function of pumping what is necessary for the circulation of blood. It is the most massive part of the heart.

- *Endocardium* – This is the smooth innermost layer that keeps the blood from sticking to the inside of the heart.

The heart wall is uneven because some parts of the heart – like the atria -- don't need a lot of muscle power to perform their duties. Other parts, like the ventricles, require a thicker muscle to pump the blood.

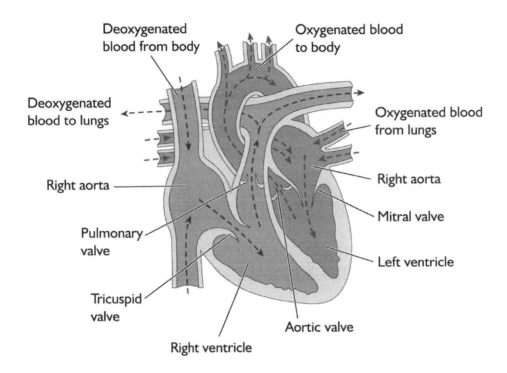

2. Four Chambers of the Heart

There are four chambers in the heart. These are:

- *Right atrium*
- *Left atrium*
- *Right ventricle*
- *Left ventricle*

The *atria* (plural for *atrium*) are smaller than the ventricles, and they have thin walls, as their function is to receive blood from the lungs and the body and pump it to the ventricles. The *ventricles* have to pump the blood to the lungs and the rest of the body, so they are larger and have a thicker wall. The left half of the heart, which is responsible for pumping the blood through the body, has a thicker wall than the right half, and this left ventricle pumps the blood to the lungs.

The blood vessels have one way valves allowing the blood to only flow in one direction. The valves that keep the blood from going back into the atria from the ventricles are called the *atrioventicular valves*, and the valves that keep the blood from going back from the arteries into the ventricles are called the *semilunar valves.*

The pumping function of the heart is made possible by two groups of cells that set the heart's pace and keep it well coordinated: the sinoatrial and the atrioventicular node.

- The *sinoatrial node* sets the pace and signals the atria to contract

- The *atrioventicular node* picks up the signal from the sinoatrial node, and this signal tells the ventricles to contract.

B. The Blood Vessels

The *blood vessels* carry the blood from the heart, to the body and then back. They vary in size depending on the amount of the blood that needs to flow through them. The hollow part in the middle, called the lumen, is where the blood actually flows. The vessels are lined with *endothelium,* which is made out of the same type of cells as the endocardium and serves the same purpose, to keep the blood from sticking to the walls and clotting.

1. Arteries

Arteries are blood vessels that transport the blood away from the heart. They work under a lot more pressure than the other types of blood vessels; hence, they have a thicker, more muscular wall, which is also highly elastic. The smaller arteries are usually more muscular, while the larger are more elastic.

The Aorta

The largest artery in the body is called the *aorta.* It ascends from the left ventricle of the heart, arches to the back left, and descends behind the heart. Narrower arteries that branch off of main arteries and carry blood to the capillaries are called *arterioles.* The descending part of the aorta carries blood to the lower parts of the body, except for the lungs. The lungs get blood through the *pulmonary artery* that comes out of the right ventricle.

The Aortic Arch

The arching part of the aorta (called the *aortic arch)* branches into three arteries: the brachiocephalic artery, the left common artery, and the left subclavian artery.

- The *brachiocephalic artery* carries blood to the brain and head. The brachiocephalic artery divides into the *right subclavian artery,* which brings the blood to the right arm.

- The *left common carotid artery* carries blood to the brain.

- The *left subclavian artery* carries blood to the left arm.

2. Veins

Veins are blood vessels that bring the blood from to the body and then back to the heart. As they don't work under the same pressure as the arteries, they are much thinner and not as muscular or elastic. The veins also have a number of one way valves that stops the blood from going back through them.

Veins use inertia, muscle work, and gravity to get the blood to the heart. Thin veins that connect to the capillaries are called *venules.* The lungs have their own set of veins: the left and right superior and inferior pulmonary veins. These vessels enter the heart through the left atrium.

Two Main Veins

The two main veins are called the superior vena cava and the inferior vena cava.

- *The superior vena cava* – This vein ascends from the right atrium and connects to the head and neck, delivering the blood supply to these structures. The superior vena cava also connects to the arms via both subclavian and brachiocephalic veins.

- *The inferior vena cava* – This vessel descends from the right atrium, carrying the blood from the lumbar veins, gonadal veins, hepatic veins, phrenic veins, and renal veins.

The lungs have their own set of veins: the left and right superior and inferior pulmonary veins. These vessels enter the heart through the left atrium.

3. Capillaries

Capillaries are the smallest blood vessels, and the most populous in the body. They can be found in almost every tissue. They connect to arterioles on one end and the venules on the other end. Also, capillaries carry the blood very close to the cells, and thus, enable cells to exchange gasses, nutrients, and cellular waste. The walls of capillaries have to be very thin for this exchange to happen.

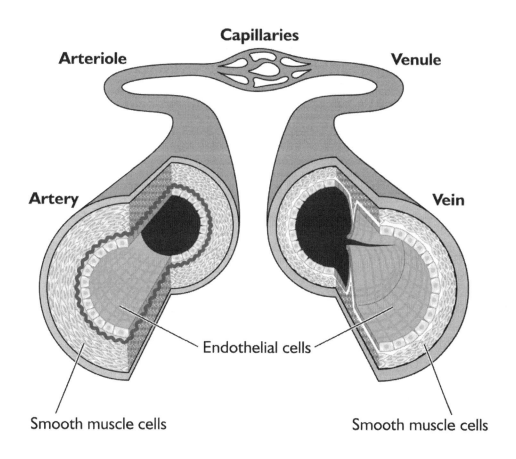

Capillaries

Arteriole

Venule

Artery

Vein

Endothelial cells

Smooth muscle cells

Smooth muscle cells

C. The Blood

The *blood* is the medium for the transport of substances throughout the body. There are 4 to 5 liters of this liquid connective tissue in the human body. The components of the blood are red blood cells, hemoglobin, white blood cells, platelets, and plasma.

1. Red Blood Cells (RBCs)

Also called erythrocytes, red blood cells (RBCs) are produced inside the red bone marrow and they serve to transport oxygen.

2. Hemoglobin (HGB)

Hemoglobin (HGB) is a red pigment found in the red blood cells, and HGB is rich in iron and proteins, which both allow these cells to transport the oxygen. Hemoglobin also has a biconcave shape, which means it is round and thinner in the middle. This shape gives them a larger surface area, making them more effective.

3. White blood cells (WBCs)

Also called leukocytes, white blood cells (WBCs) are important for the human immune system. There are two classes of white blood cells: granular and agranular leukocytes.

4. **Platelets** Also called thrombocytes, platelets are vital   for blood clotting. They are formed in the red bone marrow and serve many functions in the body.

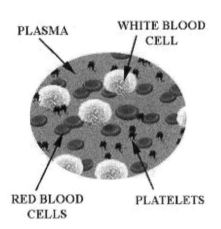

5. **Plasma** The plasma is the liquid part of the blood, and it forms 55 percent of the total blood volume. Plasma consists of up to 90 percent water, as well as proteins – Including antibodies and albumins. Other substances in plasma are circulating in the blood plasma, also, such as glucose, nutrients, cell waste, and various gasses.

- Granular leukocytes are divided into three types: the neutrophils that digest bacteria, the eosinophils that digest viruses, and the basophils that release histamine.

- Agranular leukocytes are divided into two classes: the lymphocytes, which fight off viral infections and produce antibodies for fighting pathogen-induced infection and the monocytes, which play a role in removing pathogens and dead cells from wounds.

D. Physiology of the Heart and the Circulatory System

The heart works by shifting between two states: systole and diastole.

- Systole means the cardiac muscles are contracting and moving blood from any given chamber

- Diastole means the muscles are relaxing and the chamber is expanding to fill with blood.

The systole and diastole are responsible for the pressure in the major arteries. This is the blood pressure that is measured in a regular exam. The two values are systolic and diastolic pressures respectively, with the former being larger than the latter.

1. The Cardiac Cycle

A cardiac cycle is a series of events that happen during one heartbeat. These events include:

1. Atrial systole – The first phase of the cardiac cycle is atrial systole. With this, the blood is pushed by the atria through the valves into ventricles, which are in diastole during that event.

2. Ventricular systole – After atrial systole, ventricular systole occurs. This pushes the blood from the ventricles to the organs, which occurs while the atria are in diastole.

3. Relaxation phase – After ventricular systole, there is a pause called the relaxation phase. During this, all the chambers are in diastole, and the blood enters the atria through the veins.

4. Refilling phase – When atria are at about 75 percent of their capacity, the cycle starts again. With the refilling phase, the atria are fully filled before atrial systole occurs again.

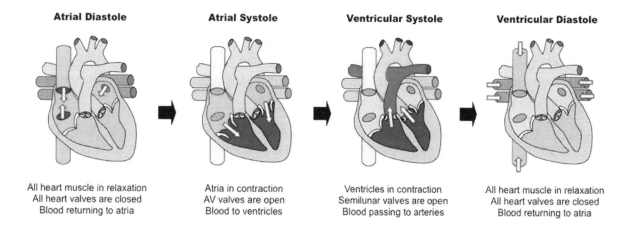

Atrial Diastole

All heart muscle in relaxation
All heart valves are closed
Blood returning to atria

Atrial Systole

Atria in contraction
AV valves are open
Blood to ventricles

Ventricular Systole

Ventricles in contraction
Semilunar valves are open
Blood passing to arteries

Ventricular Diastole

All heart muscle in relaxation
All heart valves are closed
Blood returning to atria

2. Oxygenating the Blood Cells

There are four steps to blood cell oxygenation. These include:

1. The poorly oxygenated blood comes into the right atrium through the superior and inferior vena cava.

2. The blood is then passed to the right ventricle, which sends it through the pulmonary artery into the lungs where oxygenation occurs.

3. The oxygen-rich blood then comes to the left atrium through the pulmonary veins, and gets moved from the left atrium to the left ventricle.

4. By way of blood pressure, the blood is then sent from the left ventricle through the aorta and the aortic arch into the arteries in the whole body.

Returning the Blood to the Heart

The blood passes from the arteries to the arterioles, and on from those vessels to the capillaries. The capillaries are where the exchange of gasses, nutrients, wastes, and hormones occur. The blood then passes into venules, and gets back to the heart through the veins. This way, a healthy resting heart can pump around 5 liters per minute.

The veins of the stomach and intestines don't carry the blood directly to the heart. Rather, they divert it to the liver first, through the hepatic portal vein, so that the liver can store sugar, remove toxins, and process the products of digestion. The blood then goes to the heart through the inferior vena cava.

These processes enable the circulatory system to perform its role of transportation, protection, and regulation. Using the cardiovascular and pulmonary systems, the body transports nutrients, gasses, cellular waste, and hormones. The blood also helps with temperature regulation and homeostasis.

Circulatory Questions:

1. At what rate does a healthy heart pump blood while resting?

    a) Around 3 liters per minute.
    b) Around 8 liters per minute.
    c) Around 5 liters per minute.

2. Which of the layers of the wall of the heart contains cardiac muscles?

    a) Myocardium
    b) Epicardium
    c) Endocardium

3. The heart chamber with the thickest wall is:

    a) The left ventricle
    b) The right ventricle
    c) The right atrium

4. The blood from the left ventricle goes to:

    a) The right ventricle
    b) The vena cava
    c) The aorta and aortic arch

5. The blood vessels that carry the blood from the heart are called:

    a) Veins
    b) Arteries
    c) Capillaries

6. Blood is prevented from changing direction in the veins by:

    a) Pressure from the heart
    b) Valves
    c) Suction from the heart

7. The liquid part of the blood is called:

    a) Plasma
    b) Blood fluid
    c) Serous fluid

8. Blood cells that are responsible for transportation of oxygen are called:

    a) Leukocytes
    b) Thrombocytes
    c) Erythrocytes

9. When measuring blood pressure, the numbers represent:

    a) The systolic and diastolic pressures, respectively.
    b) The diastolic and systolic pressures, respectively.
    c) The pressure in the arteries and the veins, respectively.

10. The superior vena cava:

    a) Ascends from the right atrium.
    b) Ascends from the left atrium.
    c) Descends from the right atrium.

The Cardiovascular System ANSWERS

    1. C)
    2. A)
    3. A)
    4. C)
    5. B)
    6. B)
    7. A)
    8. C)
    9. A)
    10. A)

The Respiratory System

The human body needs oxygen in order to function. The system that is responsible for intake of the gas is called the respiratory system. It's also in charge of removing carbon dioxide from the body, which is equally important. The respiratory system can be divided into two sections: the upper respiratory tract and the lower respiratory tract.

A.   The Upper Respiratory Tract

The *upper respiratory tract* consists of the nose, nasal cavity, olfactory membranes, mouth, pharynx, epiglottis, and the larynx.

1. The Nose
The nose is the primary body part for air intake and removing carbon dioxide. The nose itself is made out of bone, cartilage, muscle, and skin, and it serves as a protector of the hollow space behind it called the nasal cavity.

2. The Nasal Cavity
The nasal cavity is covered with hair and mucus, which together serve an important function – they stop contaminants from the outside. Common contaminants include dust, mold, and other particles. The nasal cavity permits the contaminants from entering further into the respiratory system. The three important roles of the nasal cavity are:

- Moisturizing
- Warming
- Filtering the air

3. Olfactory Membranes
The nose and the nasal cavity also contain olfactory membranes, which are small organs responsible for our sense of smell. They are located on the top of the nasal cavity, just under the bridge of the nose.

4. The Mouth
We can also breathe through the mouth, although it is not the primary breathing opening. The mouth doesn't perform as well when it comes to the three functions of the primary opening: filtering, moisturizing, and warming of air. However, the mouth does have its advantages over the nose when it comes to breathing. These advantages include:

175

- It is larger than the nose and can take in a larger amount of air.

- It is physically closer to the lungs, making the passage of air shorter.

- That's why we breathe through the mouth when we need a lot of air fast.

5. The Pharynx (Throat)

The next part of the respiratory system is the throat, which is also called the pharynx. The pharynx is a smooth, muscular structure. It is lined with mucous that is divided into three regions:

- The nasopharynx

- The oropharynx

- The laryngopharynx

The air comes in through the nose, and then passes through the *nasopharynx,* which is also where the Eustachian tubes from the middle ears connect with the pharynx. The air continues through the rest of the throat and then comes in through the mouth. Once air enters the throat, it is in the oropharynx, which is the same passageway used for transporting food when eating. Both air and food also pass through the laryngopharynx, which is where these substances get diverted.

6. Epiglottis

The body part that is responsible for keeping air going into the trachea and the food going into the esophagus is called epiglottis. The epiglottis is a flap made of elastic cartilage, which covers the opening of one passage way to allow the air or food to go into the other one. When breathing, the opening of the esophagus is covered, and when swallowing, the opening of the trachea is covered.

7. The Larynx (Voice Box)

The larynx is the part of the airway that sits between the pharynx and the trachea. It is also called the voice box, because it contains mucous membrane folds that vibrate when air passes through them to produce vocal sounds – the vocal folds. The larynx is made out of several cartilage structures:

- The epiglottis

- The thyroid cartilage - Known as the Adam's apple

- The cricoid cartilage – Which is a ring-shaped structure that keeps the larynx open.

B.   The Lower Respiratory Tract

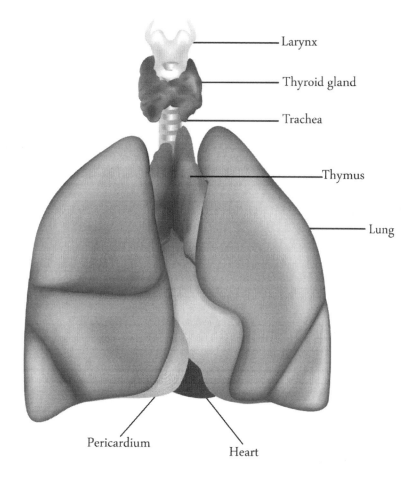

The *lower respiratory tract* – This consists of the trachea, bronchi, lungs, and the muscles that help with breathing.

1.   Trachea (Windpipe)

The *lower respiratory tract* begins with the *trachea,* also known as the windpipe. The trachea is the part of the respiratory system between the larynx and the bronchi. As its name suggest, the windpipe resembles a pipe, and it's really flexible so it can follow various head and neck movements. The trachea is made out of fibrous and elastic tissues, smooth muscle, and about 20 cartilage rings.

The interior of the windpipe is lined with mucus-producing cells, as well as cells that have small fringes that resemble hair. These hair-like structures (cilia) allow the air to pass through the windpipe, where it is further filtered by the mucous. Also, the fringes help with moving the mucous up the airways and out, to keep the air passage free.

177

2. Bronchi

Connecting to the trachea are the *bronchi,* which branch to the left and the right of the primary bronchi to be precise. The primary bronchi are made out of many C-shaped cartilage rings, and they branch into the secondary bronchi. Two of them branch from the left primary bronchi, and three branch from the right, corresponding to the number of lobes in the lungs.

The secondary bronchi contain less cartilage and have more space between the rings. The same goes for the tertiary bronchi into which the secondary bronchi are divided in the lobes of the lungs. All of the bronchi are lined with *epithelium* that contains:

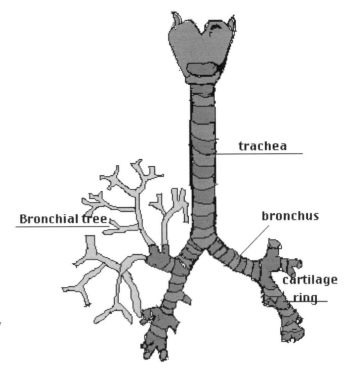

* The *goblet cells* – These produce the mucus that coats the lining of the bronchi and traps foreign particles and organisms, and
* The *cilia* – These are hair-like structures that move the mucus up and out of the lungs, keeping them clean and healthy.

3. Bronchioles

Bronchioles branch from the tertiary bronchi. They contain no cartilage at all; rather, they are made of smooth muscle and elastic fiber tissue, which allows them to be quite small and still able to change their diameter. Bronchioles end with terminal bronchioles, which connect them with alveoli. The changes that occur include:

* When the body needs more oxygen, they expand
* When there is a danger of pollutants entering the lungs, they constrict.

4. Alveoli

Alveoli are where the gas exchange happens. Alveoli are small cavities located in alveolar sacs and surrounded by capillaries. The inner surface of alveoli is coated with alveolar fluid, which plays a vital role in keep the alveoli moist, the lungs elastic, and the thin wall of alveoli stable.

The wall of the alveoli is made out of alveolar cells and the connective tissue which forms the respiratory membrane where it comes in contact with the wall of the capillaries.

5. The Lungs

The lungs themselves are two spongy organs that contain the bronchi, bronchioles, alveoli, and blood vessels. The lungs are contained in the rib cage, and are surrounded by the pleura, a double-layered membrane. The pleura consist of:

* The outer layer, called the parietal pleura.

- The inner layer, called the visceral pleura.

Between the layers of the pleura is a hollow space called the pleural cavity, which allows the lungs to expand. The lungs are wider at the top, which is referred to as the base, and they are narrower at the bottom part, which is called the apex. The lungs are divided into lobes, with the larger lung – the right one – consisting of three lobes, and the smaller lung – the left lung – consisting of two lobes.

6. **The Muscles of Respiration**

The muscles that play a major role in respiration are the diaphragm and the intercostal muscles. The diaphragm is a structure made of skeletal muscle, and it located under the lungs, forming the floor of the thorax. The intercostal muscles are located between the ribs. There are two types of intercostal muscles:

- The internal intercostal muscles – These help with breathing out (expiration) by depressing the ribs and compressing the thoracic cavity.
- The external intercostal muscles – These do the opposite and help with breathing in (inspiration).

C. Physiology of the Lungs and the Respiratory System

Breathing in and out is also called pulmonary ventilation. The two types of pulmonary ventilation are inhalation and exhalation.

1. **Inhalation – Inspiration**

- The diaphragm contracts and moves a few inches towards the stomach, making more space for the lungs to expand, and this movement pulls the air into the lungs.
- The external intercostal muscles also contract to expand the rib cage, and pull more air into the lungs.
- The lungs are naturally at a pressure lower than the atmosphere, or negative pressure, which also makes air come into to lungs until reaching a certain point. At this point, the pressure inside the lungs and the atmospheric pressure are the same.
- The diaphragm and the external intercostal muscles then expand the thoracic cavity to make the pressure in the lungs below that of the atmosphere, and this action continues to fill the lungs with air.

2. **Exhalation – Expiration**

- When breathing out, the diaphragm and the external intercostal muscles relax, and the internal intercostal muscles contract.
- The thoracic cavity becomes smaller, and the pressure in the lungs gets higher than the atmospheric pressure, which moves air out of the lungs.
- After this, the lungs return back to the negative pressure state by themselves.

3. **Different Types of Breathing**

Shallow breathing is one type of ventilation where air is moved at around half of a liter. This is called tidal volume. During deep breathing, a larger amount of air is moved (three to five liters), and this is known as vital capacity. The abdominal and other muscles are also involved in breathing in and out during deep breathing.

Eupnea is a term for the breathing our body does when resting, which consists of mostly shallow breaths, with an occasional deep breath. The lungs are never completely without air – around a liter of air is always present in the lungs.

Respiratory Questions:

1. The primary opening for breathing in and out is:

   a) The nose
   b) The mouth
   c) The skin pores

2. The air that we breathe in through the mouth enters the throat at the:

   a) Nasopharynx
   b) Oropharynx
   c) Laryngopharynx

3. For the air to go the lungs, the epiglottis needs to close:

   a) The esophagus
   b) The pharynx
   c) The larynx

4. How many lobes does the left lung have?

   a) 3
   b) 4
   c) 2

5. Bronchioles branch from the:

   a) Primary bronchi
   b) Secondary bronchi
   c) Tertiary Bronchi

6. What is the thyroid cartilage commonly known as?

   a) Vocal box
   b) Adams apple
   c) Vocal cords

7. When breathing out, the diaphragm:

   a) Relaxes
   b) Contracts
   c) Does nothing

8. Where are the cilia found?

    a) In the bronchi
    b) In the alveoli
    c) In the upper airways

The Respiratory System ANSWERS

    1. A)
    2. B)
    3. A)
    4. C)
    5. C)
    6. B)
    7. A)
    8. A)

The Skeletal System

There are a number of roles the skeletal system plays in the body. The bones and joints that make the skeletal system are responsible for:

- Providing support and protection.
- Allowing movement.
- Blood cell genesis.
- Storing fat, iron, and calcium.
- Guiding the growth of the entire body.

Generally, the skeleton can be divided into two divisions: the axial skeleton and the appendicular skeleton.

- The axial skeleton - Consists of 80 bones, which are placed along the body's midline axis and grouped into the regions of skull, ribs, and sternum as well as the vertebral column.
- The appendicular skeleton - Consists of 126 bones grouped into the regions of upper and lower limbs, as well as the pelvic and the pectoral girdle.

A. Bone Components

1. Bone Parts

On the cellular level, the bone consists of two distinctively different parts: the matrix and living bone cells.

- The bone matrix – This is the non-living part of the bone, which is made out of water, collagen, protein, calcium phosphate, and calcium carbonate crystals.
- The living bone cells – These are found at the edges of the bones and throughout the bone matrix in small cavities. Bone cells play a vital part in the growth, development, and repair of bones, and can be used for the minerals they store.

2. Bone Layers

A cross section of a bone reveals that it is made out of layers. These include:

- Periosteum – This is the topmost layer of the bone, and it is a layer of connective tissue on the surface of the bones. The periosteum contains collagen fibers that serve to anchor the tendons and the muscles, as well as the stem and the osteoblast cells that are necessary for growth and repair of the bones. Nervous tissue, nerve endings, and blood vessels are also present in the periosteum.

- Compact bone – Under the periosteum is a layer of compact bone, which gives the bone its strength. Made out of mineral salts and collagen fibers, it also contains many cavities where the living bone cells - osteocytes - can be found.

- Trabeculae – Under the compact bone is a layer where the bone tissue grows in columns called trabeculae. The bone tissue forms space that contains the red bone marrow. The trabeculae give the bone structural strength by the way they grow, while keeping them light.

B. The Five Types of Bones
The five types of bones are:

- Long
- Short
- Flat
- Irregular
- Sesamoid

1. Long Bones
The long bones make up the major bones of the limbs. They are longer than they are wide, and they are responsible for the most of our height. The long bones can be divided in two regions: the epiphyses, located at the ends of the bone, and diaphysis, located in the middle. The middle of the diaphysis contains a hollow medullary cavity, which serves as a storage for bone marrow.

2. The Short Bones
The short bones are roughly as long as they are wide, and are generally cube-shaped or round. Short bones in the body include the carpal bones of the wrist and tarsal bones of the foot.

3. The Flat Bones
The flat bones do not have the medullary cavity because they are thin and usually thinner on one end regions. Flat bones in the body include the ribs, the hip bones, as well as the frontal, the parietal, and the occipital bones of the skull.

4. The Irregular Bones
The irregular bones are those bones that do not fit the criteria to be the long, the short, or the flat bones. The vertebrae and the sacrum, among others, are irregular bones.

5. The Sesamoid Bones
There are only two sesamoid bones that are actually counted as bones: the patella and the pisiform bone. Sesamoid bones are formed inside the tendons located across the joints, and apart from the two mentioned, they are not present in all people.

C. The Joints

The joints, also known as articulations, are where the bones come into contact with each other, the cartilage, or the tooth. There are three types of joints: synovial, fibrous, and cartilaginous joints.

1. Synovial Joints

The synovial joints feature a small gap between the bones that is filled with synovial fluid, which lubricates the joint. They are the most present type of joints in the body, and they allow the most of the movement.

2. Fibrous Joints

The fibrous joints enable little to no movement, as they are present where the bones fit tight together. These joints also hold the teeth in their sockets.

3. Cartilaginous Joints

The cartilaginous joints enable little movement, as they're present where there is a layer of cartilage between two bones. They also are present where the bones meet the cartilage.

D. The Skull

Made out of 22 bones, the skull protects the brain and the sense organs for vision, hearing, smell, taste and balance. The skull has only one movable joint that connects it with the mandible – the jaw bone, which is the only movable bone of the skull. The other 21 are fused together.

1. Cranium

The upper part of the skull is known as the cranium, which is the part that protects the brain, while the lower and frontal parts of the skull form the facial bones.

2. Hyoid

Located just under the mandible, and not a part of the skull, is the hyoid bone. The hyoid is the only bone in the body that is not attached to any other bone. It helps with keeping the trachea open, and is where the tongue muscles are anchored.

3. Auditory Ossicles

Another group of bones that are not a part of the skull, but are closely connected are the auditory ossicles: the malleus, incus and stapes. They play an important role in hearing.

E. The Vertebral Column

The vertebral column, or the spine, begins at the base of the skull and stretches through the trunk down the middle and to the back to the coccyx. It is made out of 24 vertebrae, plus the sacrum and the coccyx – the tailbone.

1. Three Vertebrae Groups

The 24 vertebrae are divided into three groups:

- The cervical, or the neck vertebrae – 7 of them
- The thoracic, or the chest vertebrae – 12 of them
- The lumbar, or the lower back vertebrae – 5 of them

Furthermore, each vertebra has its own name, which is devised from the first letter of the group it belongs (for example, L for lumbar vertebrae). The letter is placed in the group, followed by a number (the first of the lumbar vertebrae is thus called L1). The spine provides support for the weight of the upper body, allows for us to maintain posture and to move, and protects the spinal cord.

VERTEBRAL COLUMN

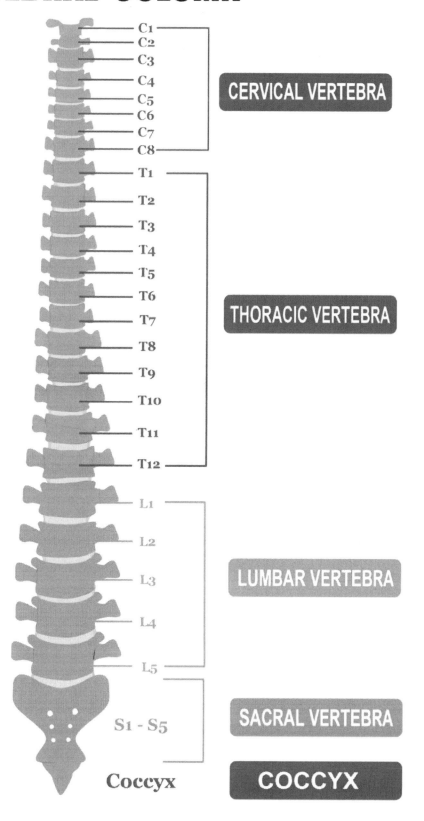

C1
C2
C3
C4
C5
C6
C7
C8

CERVICAL VERTEBRA

T1
T2
T3
T4
T5
T6
T7
T8
T9
T10
T11
T12

THORACIC VERTEBRA

L1
L2
L3
L4
L5

LUMBAR VERTEBRA

S1 - S5

SACRAL VERTEBRA

Coccyx

COCCYX

F. The Ribs and the Sternum

The ribs and the sternum are the bones that form the rib cage of the thoracic region. The sternum is also known as the breastbone. It is a thin bone that goes along the midline of the thoracic region, and most of the ribs are connected to this bone via the costal cartilage, a thin band of cartilage.

There are 12 ribs altogether. On the back side, they are attached to the thoracic vertebrae. On the front, first 7 of them attach directly to the sternum, the next 3 attach to the cartilage between the seventh rib and the sternum, and the remaining 2 do not attach to the sternum at all. Rather, they protect the kidneys, not the lungs and heart. The first 7 ribs are known as the true ribs, and the rest are known as false ribs.

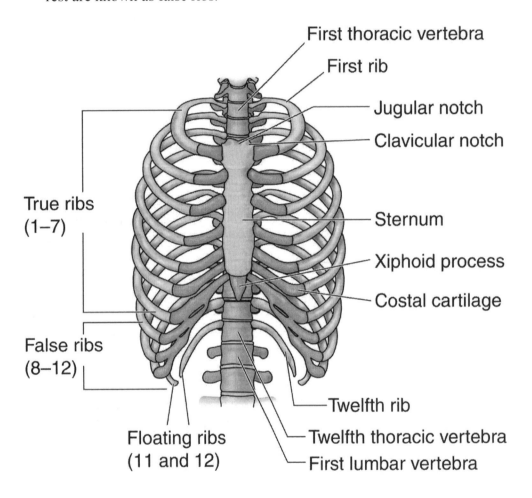

G. The Upper Limbs

The upper limbs, which belong to the appendicular skeleton, are connected with the axial skeleton by the pectoral girdle. The pectoral girdle is formed from the left and right clavicle and scapula. The scapula and the humerus, the bones of the upper arm, form the ball and socket of the shoulder joint. On its other end, the humerus forms the elbow joint.

1. **Two Forearm Bones**

   - The ulna – This bone forms the elbow joint with the humerus.
   - The radius – This bone allows the turning movement at the wrist.

2. **The Wrist Bones**
   The wrist joint is formed out of the forearm bones and the 8 carpal bones, which themselves are connected with the 5 metacarpal bones. Together, these structures form the bones of the hand. The metacarpals connect with the fingers, each made out of 3 bones called phalanges, except the thumb which only has 2 phalanges.

H. The Lower Limbs

The lower limbs, which belong to the appendicular skeleton just like the upper limbs, are connected to the axial skeleton by the pelvic girdle. The pelvic girdle is made out of the left and right hip bone.

1. **The Hip Bones**
   The hip joint is formed by the hip bone and the femur, which is the largest bone in the body. On its other end, the femur forms the knee joint with the patella – the kneecap – and the tibia, which is one of the bones of the lower leg.

2. **Leg Bones**
   Out of the two lower leg bones, the tibia is the larger one, and it serves to carry to weight of the body. The fibula, the other one, serves mostly to anchor the muscle. Together, these two bones form the ankle joint with one of the 7 tarsal bones of the foot, called the talus.

3. **Foot Bones**
   The tarsal bones form the back part of the foot and the heel. They connect to the 5 long metatarsals, which form the foot itself and connect to the toes. Each toe is made out of 3 phalanges, except the big toe, which has only 2 phalanges.

I. Physiology of the Skeletal System

The fact that the bones are connected by joints, and that they serve as anchor points for muscles, means these structures are vital for movement. The support and protection role of the skeletal system can be seen within every part group of bones:

- The skull protects and supports the brain and sensor organs.
- The thoracic cage supports and protects the lungs and heart.
- The vertebral column supports the upper body while protecting the spinal column.
- The limbs provide support and they serve as anchor points for muscles.

1. **Hematopoiesis and Calcification**

   Inside the red bone marrow, which is located in the medullar cavity of the bones, a process called hematopoiesis occurs. In the process, white and red blood cells are made. The amount of the red bone marrow declines at the end of puberty, as a significant part of it is replaced by the yellow bone marrow.

   When we are born, we have 300 bones. As we grow, the structure of the bones changes. The bones change their structure – from mostly hyaline cartilage and connective tissue to the osseous tissue – in the process called calcification. They also fuse together, which is why adults have 206 instead of 300 bones.

Skeletal System Questions:

1. How many bones do adults have?

   a) 201
   b) 300
   c) 206

2. The stem cells can be found in the:

   a) Red bone marrow
   b) Periosteum
   c) Compact bone

3. The long bones are the main bones of the:

   a) Limbs
   b) Thoracic cage
   c) Scull

4. The jaw bone is called the:

   a) Mandible
   b) Cranium
   c) Hyoid

5. The second vertebra in the chest region is called:

   a) L2
   b) T3
   c) T2

6. Which bone forms the rib cage of the thoracic region with the ribs?

   a) Sternum
   b) Fibula
   c) Occipital bone

7. The humerus and ulna form the:

   a) Shoulder joint
   b) Elbow joint
   c) Writs joint

8. Patella is also called:

    a) Breastbone
    b) Kneecap
    c) Finger bone

The Skeletal System ANSWERS

    1. C)
    2. B)
    3. A)
    4. A)
    5. C)
    6. A)
    7. B)
    8. B)

The Muscular System

Movement is the main function of the muscular system. Muscles can be found attached to the bones in our bodies, but they are also present in the heart, the blood vessels, and digestive organs. The muscles also help movement, but not of the body itself. Instead, they facilitate movement of substances through the body.

There are three types of muscle:

- Visceral muscle
- Cardiac muscle
- Skeletal muscle

A. Visceral Muscle

Visceral muscle, also known as smooth muscle, is the weakest type of muscle. It can be found in the stomach, intestines, and blood vessels, where it helps contract and move substances through them. We cannot consciously control visceral muscles – they are controlled by the unconscious part of the brain. That's why it's sometimes referred to as involuntary muscle.

The term smooth muscle is given to visceral muscle because of its appearance under the microscope. The cells of the visceral muscle form a smooth surface, which is not the case with the other two types of muscle.

B. Cardiac Muscle

Cardiac muscle is only found in the heart, where it makes the heart contract and pump blood through the body. Although the heart is not controlled by the unconscious part of the brain, like visceral muscle, it is still an involuntary muscle. This is because the impulse to contract comes from the heart itself, and it's not consciously controllable.

Unlike the visceral muscle, the cardiac muscle is very strong, and when observed under a microscope, it looks like light and dark stripes. This is caused by the arrangement of protein inside the cells, which has a lot to do with its strength.

The cardiac muscle cells have to be very resistant to deal with the blood pressure, and they work constantly to pump the blood. These cells are shaped like the letters X and Y, and these branches become intertwined and form structures called intercalated disks. They keep the cells strongly bonded together, which helps with their endurance.

C. Skeletal Muscle

Skeletal muscle is the only type of muscle that contracts and relaxes by voluntary action. Skeletal muscle is attached to the bone by tendons or at least one end. Tendons are formed out of connective tissue rich in collagen fibers.

Skeletal muscle is made out of cells that are lumped together to form fiber structures. These fibers are covered by a cell membrane called the sarcolemma, which serves as a conductor for electrochemical signals that tell the muscle to contract or expand. The transverse tubes, which are connected to the sarcolemma, transfer the signals deeper, into the middle of the muscle fiber.

Calcium ions, which are necessary for contraction of the muscle, are stored in the sarcoplasmic reticulum. The fibers are also rich in mitochondria, which act as power stations fueled by sugars and providing the energy necessary for the muscle to work. Muscle fibers are mostly made out of myofibrils, which do the actual contraction, and are made out of protein fibers arranged into small subunits called sarcomeres.

1. **Two Types of Skeletal Muscle Fibers**
   Skeletal muscle can be divided into two types, according to the way they produce and use energy. These include:

   - Type I – These are slow contracting, fatigue-resistant fibers that are used for stamina and posture. They owe their fatigue resistance to the fact they produce energy from sugar using aerobic respiration.
   - Type II – These are stronger but less enduring muscles. Type II A are mostly found in legs and are less strong and more enduring than Type II B, which are found mostly in the arms.

2. **How Skeletal Muscles Work**
   Skeletal muscles work by contracting. This shortens the length in their middle part, called the muscle belly, which in turn pulls one bone closer to another. The place of the bone that is not actually moving – that remains stationary – is called the origin. The insertion is the place of the other bone, the one that is actually moving towards the other.

   Skeletal muscles rarely work alone. They usually work in groups, in which the main muscle responsible for the action is called the agonist, and it's always paired with another muscle that does the opposite action, called antagonist. If the two were to contract together at the same time, they would cancel each other out and produce no movement. Other muscles that support the agonist are:

   - Synergists – Usually found near the agonist and attached to the same bones, stabilize the movement and reduce unnecessary movement.
   - Fixators – Which keep the origin stable.

3. **Naming the Skeletal Muscles**
   With more than 600 skeletal muscles in the human body, naming them is done in several different ways. A lot of skeletal muscles are named by the region of body they can be found in, like transverse abdominis, which can be found in the region of the abdomen. They can also be named by the part of the bone they are anchored to – like the tibialis anterior.

   Skeletal muscles are also named by the number of origins, since skeletal muscles that connect to more than one bone, or to more places on a single bone, have a larger number of origins. These are called:

- Biceps – They have two origins.
- Triceps – Which have three origins.
- Quadriceps – With four origins.

The easiest way to find muscles is by origin and insertion, because they get their name from the bones they are attached. For instance, the occipitofrontalis is attached to the occipital and the frontal bones.

Skeletal muscles can also be named by their function, like the flexor muscles of the forearm, which flex the wrist and fingers. Also, the deltoid muscle is named by its shape. Some muscles are named by the direction of the muscle fiber that makes them. Obliques are thus named because their muscle fiber runs at an angle.

When there are a number of similar muscles in the same region that vary in size, the largest is called the maximus, the middle one is called the medius, and the smallest is named the minimus. For example, the gluteus group: the gluteus maximus, gluteus medius, and gluteus minimus.

D. Physiology of the Muscular System

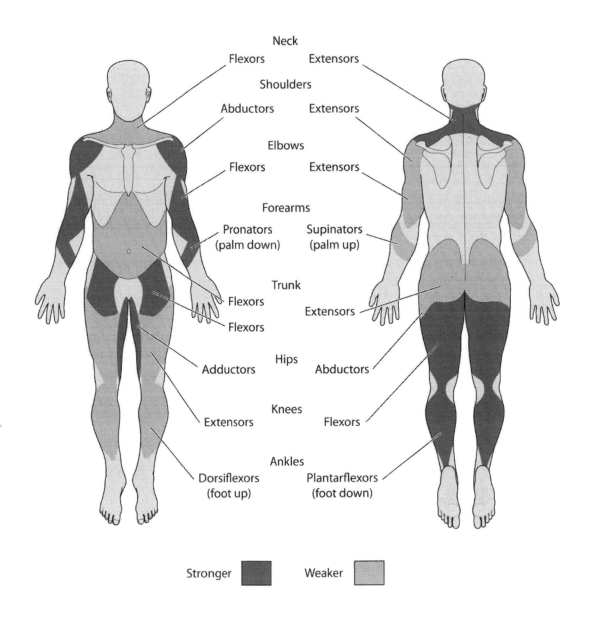

The muscular system has four functions:

- Movement – It enables us to move.
- Maintaining the posture – It enables us to stand still or in a particular position.
- Substance movement through the body – this is the main role of the cardiac and visceral muscles.
- Body heat generation – When muscles work, they produce a lot of waste heat, which is responsible for our natural body temperature as well as the raised temperature after exertion.

1. **Motor Neurons and Units**

   The neurons that control the muscles are called the motor neurons. These control a number of muscle cells that are called the motor unit. The number of cell in the motor unit is larger in large muscles that need more strength, like the muscles in the arms and legs. In small muscles that need precision more than strength, like the muscles in the fingers and around the eyes, the number of cells in motor units is smaller.

2. **Types of Contractions**

   There are a number of different muscle contractions:

   - Isotonic muscle contractions – These are muscle contractions that produce movement.
   - Isometric muscle contractions – This type does not produce movement; rather, they maintain posture and keep us still.
   - Muscle tone – This involves naturally occurring constant semi contraction of the muscle.
   - Twitch contraction – This is a short contraction caused by a single, short nerve impulse.
   - Temporal summation – This is a phenomenon in which a few short impulses delivered over time build up the muscle contraction in strength and duration.
   - Tetanus – This is a state of constant contraction caused by many rapid short impulses.

3. Muscle Metabolism
Two Ways Muscles Get Energy

There are two ways for the muscle to get energy:

- Using oxygen from aerobic respiration, which is the more effective way to get energy.
- Using lactic acid fermentation, which is a type of anaerobic respiration. It's less effective and it only happens when the blood cannot get into the muscle due to the very strong contraction.

Both of these methods are aimed at producing adenosine tri-phosphate (ATP) from glucose. ATP is the most important energy molecule for our bodies. During its conversion adenosine di-phosphate (ADP), energy is released.

Molecules for Energy Production

Muscles also use other molecules to help in the production of energy:

- Myoglobin works similarly as hemoglobin – It stores oxygen, giving the muscles an amount of time of aerobic respiration even when there is no blood coming into the muscles.
- Creatine phosphate – Which gives its phosphate group to the energy-depleted adenosine di-phosphate and turns in back into the energy rich ATP.
- Glycogen – A large molecule made out of a number of glucose molecules. Muscles use the glucose to get ATP.

When it runs out of energy, a muscle goes into a state of muscle fatigue. This means it contains little to no oxygen, ATP, or glucose, and a lot of lactic acid and ADP. When a muscle is fatigued, it needs a lot of oxygen to replace the oxygen used from myoglobin, and to rebuild the other energy supplies.

Muscular System Questions:

1. Which type of muscle is found in the blood vessels?

   a) Cardiac muscle
   b) Skeletal muscle
   c) Visceral muscle

2. Cardiac muscle is:

   a) Involuntary muscle
   b) Voluntary muscle
   c) Both

3. Tendons attach the skeletal muscle at:

   a) Only one end always
   b) Both ends always
   c) At least one end

4. Myofibrils form:

   a) The layer around the muscle
   b) The muscle fiber
   c) The tendons

5. Which is the strongest type of skeletal muscle?

   a) Type II A
   b) Type II B
   c) Type I

6. The bone that is stationary during the movement is called the:

   a) Insertion
   b) Agonist
   c) Origin

7. How many origins does a quadriceps have?

   a) 4
   b) 5
   c) 3

8. What are the motor units made of?

a) Motor neurons
b) Muscle cells
c) Tendons

The Muscular System ANSWERS

1. C)
2. A)
3. C)
4. B)
5. B)
6. C)
7. A)
8. B)

The Nervous System

The nervous system is made out of the brain, the spinal cord, the nerves, and the sensory organs. This system is responsible for gathering, processing, and reacting to information from both within and outside of the body. It is divided into two parts: the central nervous system and the peripheral nervous system. The nervous system is mostly made out of nervous tissue, which is in turn made out of two classes of cells: the neurons and the neuralgia.

The central nervous system (CNS) is made of the brain and spinal cord and is responsible for processing and storing information, as well as deciding on the appropriate action and issuing commands.

The peripheral nervous system (PNS) is responsible for gathering information, transporting it to the CNS, and then transporting the commands from the CNS to the appropriate organs. Sensory organs and nerves do the gathering and transporting of information, while the efferent nerves transport the commands.

A. The Neurons

Neurons are the nerve cells. They can be divided into several different parts:

- The soma – This is the body of the neuron, and it contains most of the cellular organelles.
- The dendrites – These are small treelike structures that extend from the soma. Their main responsibility is to carry information to the soma, and sometimes away from it.
- The axon – This is a long, thin projection that also extends from the soma. There is usually one axon per soma, but it can branch out further down its length. It is responsible for sending information from the soma and rarely to it.
- Synapses – The places where two neurons meet, or where they meet other types of cells, are called synapses.

1. The Three Classes of Neurons

Neurons can be divided into three classes. These include:

- Efferent neurons – The motor neurons responsible for transmitting signals from the CNS to the effectors in the body.
- Afferent neurons – The sensory neurons responsible for transmitting signals from the receptors in the body to the CNS.
- Interneurons – The neurons that form the complex networks in the CNS. They are responsible for the integration of the signals received from the afferent neurons, and controlling the body by sending signals through the efferent neurons.

2. The Neuralgia

Neuralgia are the maintenance cells for the neurons. Neurons are so specialized for their task that they almost never reproduce. Therefore, they need the neuralgia cells, a number of which surrounds every neuron, to protect and feed them. Neuralgia are also called the glial cells.

B. The Central Nervous System

The CNS consists out of:

- The brain
- The spinal cord

Both the brain and the spinal cord are placed within cavities in protective skeletal structures. The brain is housed in the cranial cavity of the skull, and the spinal cord ins enclosed in the vertebral cavity in the spine.

Since the organs that form the CINS are very vital to our survival, they are also protected by two other important structures:

- The meninges
- The cerebrospinal fluid (CSF)

1. The Meninges

The meninges are a protective covering of the CNS that consists of three distinct layers:

- The dura mater – As its name suggests, is the most durable, outer part of the meninges. It is made out of collagen fibers-rich thick connective tissue, and it forms a space for the cerebrospinal fluid around the CNS.
- The arachnoid mater – This is the thin lining on the inner side of the dura mater. It forms many tiny fibers that connect the dura mater with the next layer – the pia mater.
- The pia mater – This is separated from the arachnoid mater by the subarachnoid space – a space filled with cerebrospinal fluid. The pia mater directly covers the surface of the brain and spinal cord, and it provides sustenance to the nervous tissue through its many blood vessels.

2. The Cerebrospinal Fluid

Found in the subarachnoid space, the cerebrospinal fluid is a clear fluid formed from blood plasma. It can be found in:

- The subarachnoid space.
- In the ventricles, the hollow spaces in the brain.
- In the central canal, a cavity found in the middle of the spinal cord.

As the CNS floats in the cerebrospinal fluid, it appears lighter than it really is. This is especially important for the brain, because the fluid keeps it from being crushed by its own weight. The floating also protects the brain and the spinal cord from shock – like sudden movements and trauma. Additionally, the CSF contains the necessary chemical substance for the normal functioning of the nervous tissue, and it serves to remove the cellular waste form the neurons.

3. The Brain And Nervous Tissue

The nervous tissue that makes up the brain is divided into two classes:

- The gray matter - Which consists mostly of interneurons that are unmyelinated, and is the tissue where the actual processing of signals happens. It is also where the connections between neurons are made.

- The white matter - Which consists mostly of myelinated neurons, and is the tissue that conducts signals to, from, and between the gray matter regions.

The brain can be divided into three distinct parts:
- The forebrain – Prosencephalon
- The midbrain – Mesencephalon
- The hindbrain – Rhombencephalon

The Prosencephalon

The forebrain consists out of two regions:
- The cerebrum
- The diencephalon

The Cerebrum

The outermost and the largest part of the brain, the cerebrum is divided through the middle by the longitudinal fissure into the left and the right hemisphere, which are further divided into four lobes each:
- Frontal
- Parietal
- Temporal
- Occipital

The surface of the cerebrum, called the cerebral cortex is made out of gray matter with characteristic grooves (sulci) and bulges (gyri). The cerebral cortex is where the actual processing happens in the cerebrum – it's responsible for the higher brain functions like thinking and using language. Under the cerebral cortex, there is a layer of white matter, which connects the regions of the cerebrum with one another, and the cerebrum itself with the rest of the body. It contains a special band of white matter that connects the two hemispheres, which is called the corpus callosum.

The several regions located under the white matter are divided into two groups:
- The basal nuclei, which help control and regulate the movement of muscles.
- The limbic system, which play a role in memory, emotions and survival.

The Diencephalon

The diencephalon is a structure formed by:
- The thalamus – Made out of two gray matter masses, the thalamus is located around the third ventricle of the brain. Its role is to route the sensory signals to the correct parts of the cerebral cortex.
- The hypothalamus – Located under the thalamus, the hypothalamus plays a role in regulating hunger, thirst, blood pressure and body temperature changes, as well as the heart rate and the production of hormones.

- The pineal gland – Located beneath the hypothalamus, and directly controlled by it, the pineal gland produces the hormone melatonin, which plays a vital role in sleep.

The Mesencephalon

The midbrain is the topmost part of the brain stem. It is divided into two regions:
- The tectum, which plays a role in reflex reactions to visual and auditory information
- The cerebral peduncules, which connect the cerebrum and thalamus with the lower parts of the brain stem, and the spinal cord. It also contains substantia nigra, which is involved in muscle movements by inhibiting their movements.

The Rhombencephalon

The hindbrain is made out of the brain stem and the cerebellum. The two parts of the brain stem that form the hindbrain are:
- The medulla oblongata connects the spinal cord with another part of the brainstem, called the pons. It is mostly made out of white matter, but it also contains gray matter that processes involuntary body functions like blood pressure, level of oxygen in the blood, and reflexes like sneezing, coughing, vomiting and swallowing.

- The pons are located between the medulla oblongata and the midbrain, and in front of the cerebellum. It is in charge of transporting signals to and from the cerebellum, and the between the upper regions of the brain, the medulla and the spinal cord.

The cerebellum looks like a smaller version of the cerebrum – it has two spheres and it's wrinkled. Its outer layer consists of gray matter, and it's called the cerebellar cortex, while the inner part consists of white matter which transports signals between the cerebellum and the rest of the body, and it's called the arbor vitae. The cerebellum's role is to control and coordinate complex muscle activities. It also helps us maintain posture and keep balance.

4. **The Spinal Cord**

The spinal cord, located inside the vertebral cavity, is made out of both white and gray matter. It serves to both carry signals and to process some reflexes to stimuli. The spinal nerves stretch out from it.

C. The Peripheral Nervous System

The nerves that form the peripheral nervous system are made out of bundled axons. Their role is to carry signals to and from the spinal cord and the brain. A single axon, covered with a layer of connective tissue called the endoneurium, bundles with other axons to form fascicles. These are covered with another sheath of connective tissue – the perineurium. Also, a lot of fascicles wrapped together in another layer of connective tissue – the epineurium – form a whole nerve.

1. **The Five Types of Peripheral Nerves**

There are five types of peripheral nerves:

- The afferent, efferent and mixed nerves, which are formed out of the neurons that share the same name, and they perform the same role.

- The spinal nerves – 31 pairs of them extend from the side of the spinal cord. They exit the spinal cord between the vertebrae, and they carry information to and from the spinal cord and the neck, the arms, the legs and the trunk. They are grouped and named according to the region they originate from: 8 pairs of cervical, 12 pairs of thoracic, 5 pairs of lumbar, 5 pairs of sacral, and 1 pair coccygeal nerves.
- The cranial nerves – 12 pairs of these nerves extend from the lower side of the brain. They are identified by their number, and they serve to conect the brain with the sense organs, head muscles, neck and shoulders muscle, the heart and the gastrointestinal track.

2. The Sense Organs

The sense organs include both the specialized sense organs, which are responsible for the specialized senses: the hearing, sight, balance, smell and taste. Sense organs also have sensory receptors for general senses: touch, pain and temperature. These senses are part of the PNS, and their role is to detect the stimuli and send the signal to the CNS when the detection occurs.

3. The Physiology of the Nervous System

The nervous system has three main functions:

- Sensory function is related to the intake of information from inside and outside of the body through the sensory organs and receptors, and then sending that information to the CNS.
- Integration is a process that happens in the CNS. When the signal from the sensory organs and receptors come to the CNS, the information it carries is evaluated, compared to previously stored information, stored or discarded, and used to make a decision.
- Motor function occurs once the integration is done, and the CNS may send a signal through the efferent nerves to the effector cells. These cells are located in all types of muscles and the glands, which then form a reaction to the stimuli.

The Different Divisions of the PNS

According to our ability to consciously control the PNS, it is divided into the:

- Somatic nervous system (SNS) - Which is the only part of the PNS we can consciously control. It stimulates the skeletal muscles.
- Autonomic nervous system (ANS) - Which is the part of the PNS we cannot consciously control, and which stimulates the visceral and cardiac muscle, as well as the glandular tissue.

The ANS itself is further divided into:

- The sympathetic division – Which forms the fight or flight reaction to stimuli like emotion, danger and exercise. It increases respiration and hearth rate, decreases digestion and releases stress hormones.
- The parasympathetic division – Which does the opposite of the sympathetic division after the stimuli subsides.
- Enteric nervous system (ENS) – Which is responsible for the digestive system and the processes that go on in it. This system works mostly independently from the CNS, although it can be regulated through the sympathetic and parasympathetic division.

• The Endocrine System

Another important system in our body that coordinates with the nervous system is the endocrine, or glandular, system. It controls growth rate, feelings of hunger, body temperature, and more. Many organs run the endocrine system: the pituitary gland, the pancreas, the ovaries (only in females) and testes (only in males), the thyroid gland, the parathyroid gland, the adrenal glands, etc.

Of all these, the pituitary gland is the most important endocrine gland in your body. About the size of a pea, the pituitary gland hangs down from the base of your brain and produces the hormone which controls growth.

Fun Fact: Humans grow faster at night because more hormones are released into your blood when you are sleeping.

Nervous System Questions

1. Which of the following form the CNS with the brain?

   a) The nerves
   b) The sensory organs
   c) The spinal cord

2. The part of the neuron that transports information from the cell is called:

   a) The soma
   b) The axon
   c) The dendrites

3. The motor neurons is another name for:

   a) Efferent neurons
   b) Afferent neurons
   c) Interneurons

4. The space outside the CNS filled with cerebrospinal fluid can be found:

   a) Between the dura mater and the arachnoid mater
   b) Outside the dura mater
   c) Between the arachnoid mater and the pia mater

5. The hypothalamus is located:

   a) In the mesencephalon
   b) In the rhombencephalon
   c) In the prosencephalon

6. Which part of the brain is responsible for higher brain functions?

   a) The pons
   b) The cerebral cortex
   c) The cerebellar cortex

7. How many thoracic spinal nerves are there in the human body?

   a) 8
   b) 9
   c) 12

8. Which of the following is **not** a specialized sense?

    a) Touch
    b) Balance
    c) Sight

The Nervous System ANSWERS

    1. C)
    2. B)
    3. A)
    4. C)
    5. C)
    6. B)
    7. C)
    8. A)

The Digestive System

The digestive system is a system of organs in the body that is responsible for the intake and processing of food, as well as discarding the waste products of feeding. The digestive system ensures that the body has the necessary nutrients and the energy it needs to function.

The digestive system consists of the gastrointestinal (GI) tract, which is formed by the following organs through which the food passes on its way through the body:

- The oral cavity
- The pharynx
- The esophagus
- The stomach
- The small intestines
- The large intestines

Along with the GI tract, the digestive system also contains organs that have a role in processing food, but they do not food pass through them. These include:

- The teeth
- The tongue
- The salivary glands
- The liver
- The gallbladder
- The pancreas

DIGESTIVE SYSTEM

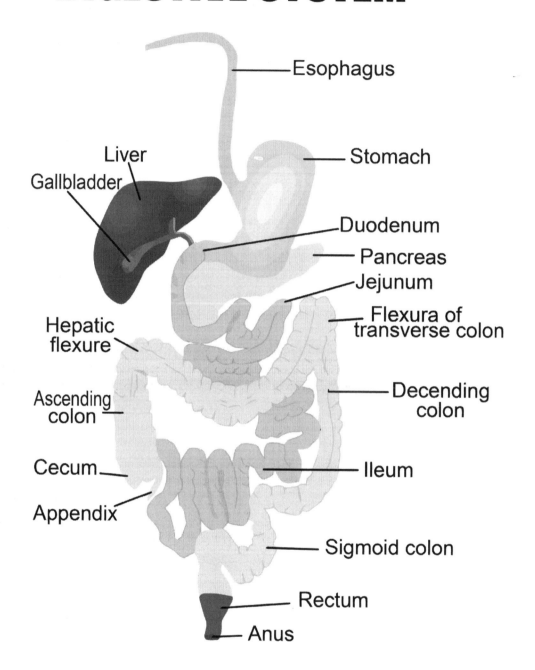

A. The Mouth

The digestive system begins with the mouth. Also known as the oral cavity, the mouth contains other organs that play a role in digestion:

- The teeth – Small organs that cut and grind food. They are located on the edges of the mouth, and are made out of dentin, which is a substance that resembles bone, and are covered by enamel. The teeth are very hard organs, and each of them has its own blood vessels and nerves, which are located in the matter that fills the tooth, called the pulp.

- The tongue – A muscle that is located in the oral cavity beneath and behind the teeth. The tongue contains the taste buds, and it plays a role in moving food around the mouth as it's being processed by the teeth and to move it towards the pharynx when it's time to swallow.
- The salivary glands – Charged with producing the saliva, these glands are located around the mouth. There are three pairs of salivary glands, and the saliva they produce serves to lubricate and digest carbohydrates.

B. The Pharynx

The pharynx is a tube that enables the passage of food and air further into the body. This structure performs two functions. The pharynx needs the help of a small flap called the epiglottis, which allows the food to pass to the esophagus by covering the opening of the larynx, a structure that carries air into the lungs. When we need to breathe in, the esophagus is closed, so the air passes only into the larynx.

C. The Esophagus

The esophagus begins at the pharynx and continues to carry food all the way to the stomach. The esophagus is a muscular tube, and the muscles in its wall help to push the food down. When throwing up, it pushes the food up.

The esophagus has two rings of muscle, called sphincters. These sphincters close at the top and the bottom ends when the food is not passing. The bottom one, when it cannot close entirely and allow the contents of the stomach to enter the esophagus, is responsible for heartburn.

D. The Stomach

The stomach is a round-shaped organ located on the left side of the body, just beneath the diaphragm. It can be divided into four different regions:

- The cardia – The region that connects with the esophagus. It is a transit from the tube-like shape of the esophagus into the sack shape of the rest of the stomach. The cardia is also where the lower sphincter of the esophagus is located.
- The body of the stomach – The largest part of the stomach.
- The fundus – Located above the body of the stomach.
- The pylorus – A funnel shaped region located beneath the body of the stomach. It controls the passage of the partially digested food further down the GI tract using the pyloric sphincter.

1. The Four Layers of Tissue in the Stomach

The stomach is made out of four layers of tissue:

- The mucosa – This is the innermost layer, which contains the mucous membrane that has a large number of cells which secrete digestive enzymes and hydrochloric acid. These cells are located within the small pores called the gastric pits. The mucous membrane also secretes a mucous that protects the stomach from its own digestive enzymes. The mucosa also contains some smooth muscle.

- The submucosa – This layer is located around the mucosa, it is made out of connective tissue and it contains the nerves and the blood vessels.
- The muscularis layer - Which as its name says, this structure is made out of three layers of smooth muscle. This layer enables the movement of the stomach.
- The serosa – This mucosa is the outermost layer. It secretes serous fluid which keeps it wet, and reduces friction between the stomach and the surrounding organs.

E. The Small Intestine

The small intestine continues from the stomach, and it takes up most of the space in the abdomen. It is around 22 feet long and looped, and it's attached to the wall of the abdomen to be kept in place.

The small intestine can be divided into three parts:

- The duodenum, which is the part of the small intestine that receives the food and chemicals from the stomach.
- The jejunum, which continues from the duodenum and is where most of the nutrients are absorbed into the blood.
- The ileum, which continues from the jejunum and where the rest of the nutrients are absorbed.

The absorption which happens in the small intestine is much helped by the villi. The villi are made out of smaller microvilli, and the villi are where the blood vessels that absorb the nutrients can be found.

F. The Liver

The liver is not a part of the GI tract. However, it performs roles that are vital for digestion and life itself. The liver is located just beneath the diaphragm, and it's the largest organ in the body after the skin. It's triangular in shape, and extends across the whole width of the abdomen.

The liver can be divided into four lobes:

- The left lobe
- The right lobe
- The caudate lobe, which wraps around the inferior vena cava
- The quadrate lobe that wraps around the gallbladder

The liver is connected to the peritoneum by four ligaments:

- The coronary ligament
- The left triangular ligament
- The right triangular ligament
- The falciform ligament

The liver is responsible for a number of different functions – from detoxification of the blood, to the storage of nutrients and production of components of blood plasma. However, for the digestive system, the role of the liver is to produce the bile, which is then carried through the bile ducts to the gallbladder.

G. The Gallbladder

Located just behind the liver, the gallbladder is a small muscular pair shaped organ. Its main role is to store bile produced by the liver and to release it into the duodenum when fat enters. This process facilitates the digestion of fat.

H. The Pancreas

The pancreas is another organ that is not a part of the GI tract, but plays a role in the digestion. It's located under the stomach and to the left. The pancreas' purpose is to secrete both the enzymes that digest the food and the hormones insulin and glucagon, which control blood sugar levels.

The pancreas is what is known as a heterocrine gland, which means it contains both the endocrine tissue, that produces insulin and glucagon, and exocrine tissue. Exocrine tissue produces:

- Pancreatic amylase - Which breaks large polysaccharides into smaller sugars
- Trypsin, chymotrypsin, and carboxypeptidase - Which break down proteins into amino acid subunits
- Pancreatic lipase - Which breaks down large fat molecules into fatty acids and monoglyceride
- Ribonuclease and deoxyribonuclease - Which digest nucleic acids.

I. The Large Intestine

The large intestine continues from the small intestine, and it surrounds its looped form. No digestion actually takes part in the large intestine. Rather, it only absorbs water and some leftover vitamins. The large intestine carries the waste (the feces) to the rectum, where it's stored until it's expelled through the anus.

J. The Digestive System Physiology

The roles of the digestive system are to:

- Ingest food
- Secrete fluids and enzymes
- Mix and move the food through the body
- Digest the food
- Absorb the food
- Remove the waste

Digestive System Review Questions:

1. The GI tract consists of:

    a) Organs of the digestive system through which the food passes
    b) Organs of the digestive system through which the food does not pass
    c) All of the organs in the digestive system

2. How many pair of salivary glands is there?

    a) 4
    b) 1
    c) 3

3. Where is the lower sphincter of the esophagus located?

    a) The body of the stomach
    b) The cardia
    c) The fundus

4. Which layer of the stomach contains the blood vessels and the nerves?

    a) The mucosa
    b) The submucosa
    c) The serosa

5. Bile is stored in:

    a) The liver
    b) The duodenum
    c) The gallbladder

6. In which region of the small intestine are most of the nutrients absorbed?

    a) The jejunum
    b) The ileum
    c) The duodenum

7. Which type of nutrients is broken down by trypsin?

    a) Proteins
    b) Fats
    c) Sugars

8. Rectum is a part of:

   a) The anus
   b) The large intestine
   c) The small intestine

The Digestive System ANSWERS

   1. A)
   2. C)
   3. B)
   4. B)
   5. C)
   6. A)
   7. A)
   8. B)

The Renal System

The renal system, also known as the urinary system, functions to remove waste products from the blood and expel them through urine. The system consists out of:

- The kidneys
- The ureters
- The urinary bladder
- The urethra

The ureters, urinary bladder and urethra together form the urinary tract, which is in charge of removing urine from the body. The kidneys, on the other hand, produce the urine.

A. The Kidneys

Located in the back of the abdominal cavity, the kidneys are a pair of bean shaped organs. On the outside, the kidneys are covered with a stiff layer of fibrous connective tissue called the renal capsule. These capsules give the kidneys their shape.

Under the renal capsule is the part of the kidney called the renal cortex, which contains a lot of blood vessels. The cortex encircles the seven cone-shaped pyramids located underneath it, which are known as the renal pyramids. Their bases are turned toward the cortex, and their apexes point away from the cortex and toward the center of the kidney.

An apex forms a connection with a small tube that serves to collect urine, called the minor calyx. These minor calyces later form the three major calyces, which merge and form the renal pelvis that extends out of the kidney itself and connects with the ureter.

ANATOMY OF THE KIDNEY

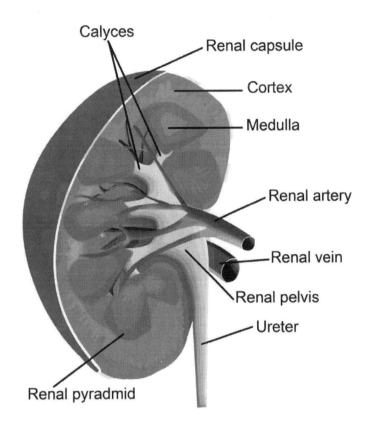

The Nephrons

The main worker cells of the kidneys are called the nephrons. They are formed out of two parts:

- The renal corpuscle, which is the part of the nephron that does the actual filtering, and which produces urine.
- The renal tubules, which carry the urine to the renal pelvis.

B. The Ureters

The ureters are two tubes that carry the urine from the kidneys and to the urinary bladder. They are 10 to 12 inches long, and they enter the urinary bladder through tunnels in its wall.

Although urine does flow down the ureters, partially because of gravity, the main force that makes it go down is actually a wave of muscle contractions in the wall of the ureters, which force the urine down.

C. The Urinary Bladder

The urinary bladder is located behind the pubic bone. Its function is to store urine. It is a muscular hollow organ that stretches as it's filled with urine coming from the ureters.

D. The Urethra

The urethra is a tube that runs from the urinary bladder and through which urine is expelled to the outer world. The wall of the urethra is lined with a mucous membrane, which contains smooth muscle and mucous glands. The mucous gland secrete mucous into the urethra.

The function of the urethra is controlled by two sphincter muscles:

- The external urethral sphincter, which is made out of skeletal muscle, allows control over when we want to urinate.
- The internal urethral sphincter, which is made out of smooth muscle, is set up to open when a certain amount of urine is present in the bladder. That's what gives us the signal that we need to urinate.

The urethra in female genitals empties into the labia minor, while in male genitals it passes through the penis, and serves as a passageway for products of reproductive system organs.

E. The Physiology of the Urinary System

The filtering role of the kidneys serves the body in more ways than one:

- Kidneys help maintain the normal level of ions and minerals in the body, as well as adjust the pH of the blood to the optimal level.
- Kidneys control how much water is filtered out of blood, which in turn keeps the cellular environment ideal for the workings of the cells in our body.
- Kidneys also help regulate the blood pressure.

The kidneys also produce hormones that interact with other systems in the body.

Renal System Questions

1. Urine is made in:
   a) The kidneys
   b) The urinary bladder
   c) The urethra
   d) None of the Above

2. Which of the following is **not** a part of the urinary tract?
   a) The urethra
   b) The left ureter
   c) The kidneys
   d) None of the Above

3. Kidneys are located in the:
   a) Front of the abdomen
   b) Back of the abdomen
   c) Middle of the abdomen
   d) None of the Above

4. What is the name of the outermost layer covering the kidney?
   a) The renal pelvis
   b) The renal cortex
   c) The renal capsule
   d) None of the Above

5. The major calyces merge to form:
   a) The renal pelvis
   b) The renal pyramids
   c) The renal cortex
   d) None of the Above

6. How many ureters are attached to a single kidney?
   a) None, they attach to the urethra
   b) 1
   c) 2
   d) None of the Above

7. The urinary bladder is located:
   a) Behind the pelvic bone
   b) In front of the pelvic bone
   c) Above the left hip bone
   d) None of the Above

8. How many sphincters control the flow of urine through urethra?
   a) 1
   b) 4
   c) 2
   d) None of the Above

The Renal System ANSWERS

   1. A)
   2. C)
   3. B)
   4. C)
   5. A)
   6. B)
   7. A)
   8. C)
   9. B)
   10. B)

The Reproductive System

The reproductive system allows humans to reproduce. The system is distinctly different in females and males.

A. The Female Reproductive System
The female reproductive system consists of:

- The ovaries
- The fallopian tubes
- The uterus
- The vagina
- The vulva
- The mammary glands
- The breasts

1. The Ovaries
The ovaries are two oval glands that are located on each side of the uterus. Within the ovaries, the female sex hormones estrogen and progesterone are produced. These hormones help the process of the eggs that can be later fertilized known as the ova.

The ova are not actually manufactured in the ovaries. Instead, they are present from birth. Out of around 60,000 eggs present at birth, only around 400 will mature during lifetime. The ovaries are attached to the uterus by the ovarian ligament, and this structure is also connected to the uterus by the fallopian tubes.

2. The Fallopian Tubes
Located between the ovaries and the uterus, the fallopian tubes are where the actual fertilization of the egg happens. When an egg is released from the ovary, it is pushed by the fimbriae, small finger like organelles that line the infundibulum. The infundibulum is the part of the tube that connects to the ovary. The egg then travels though the tube to the uterus, and is aided by the cilia and the smooth muscle of the tube.

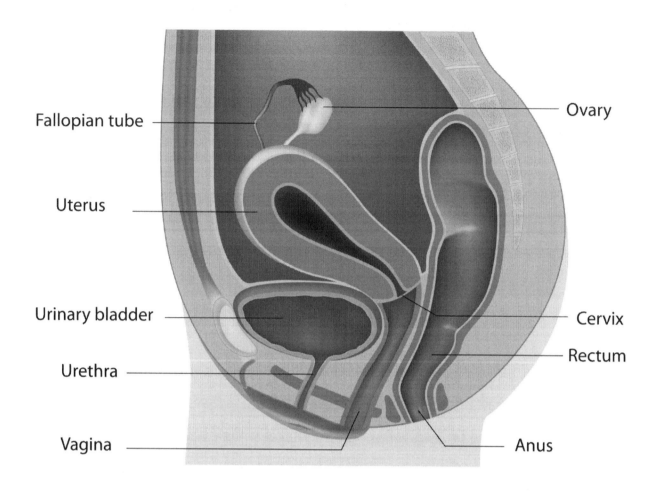

Fallopian tube

Uterus

Urinary bladder

Urethra

Vagina

Ovary

Cervix

Rectum

Anus

3. The Uterus

The uterus is a muscular, hollow organ, located above and behind the urinary bladder. It is connected to the ovaries by the fallopian tubes and to the vagina by the cervix.

The purpose of the uterus is to develop fertilized cells until they develop into an organism ready for the outside world. The uterus is lined with endometrium, a layer of tissue that helps the embryo during the earliest phases of development.

4. The Vagina

The vagina serves as a connection between the uterus and the exterior. It is located beneath the uterus, and it's shaped like a tube. The outer layer of the vagina consists of squamous epithelial tissue, which produces secretions that lubricate the vagina and make a hostile environment for bacteria, yeast, and sperm cells. This hostile environment is why the male reproduction glands produce the seminal fluid that neutralize the acidity of the secretions and ensure survival of semen.

Under the outer layer, is a layer of connective tissue rich with elastic fibers, which gives the vagina elasticity. That layer is called the lamina propria. A layer of smooth muscle cells surrounds the lamina propria, and it helps the vagina to contract and expand during intercourse and childbirth. The tunica externa, the outermost layer of the vagina, is made out of dense irregular connective tissue, and it serve as protection.

5. The Vulva

The vulva is the external genitalia. It consists of:

- The mons pubis – A layer of adipose tissue between the skin and the pubic bone.
- The labia majora – The extensions of the mons pubis.
- The labia minora – Small skin folds that are located to the inside from the labia minora, around the vaginal and urethral openings.
- The clitoris – A small mass of tissue located on the uppermost end of the labia minora, filled with nerve endings. It serves for sexual pleasure.

6. The Breast

The breasts are organs located on the left and the right sides of the thoracic region. They are made out of:

- Adipose tissue, which makes the mass of the breast.
- Milk ducts, which carry the milk.
- Mammary glands, which start producing milk during pregnancy, and stop producing it when it's no longer needed.

On the outside, the breast contains:

- The nipple, an exit for milk which is released when the nipple is stimulated.
- The areola, the darker, thicker circle surrounding the nipple, which serves to protect the inner parts breast during breastfeeding.

B. The Male Reproductive System

The male reproductive system is made out of:

- The scrotum
- The testes
- The spermatic ducts
- The sex glands
- The penis

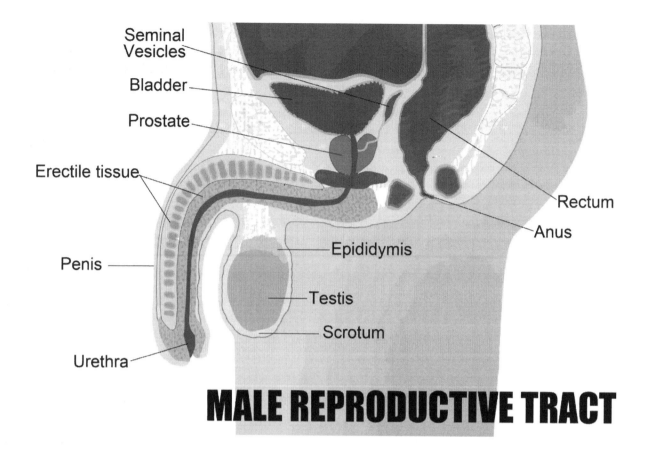

Seminal Vesicles
Bladder
Prostate
Erectile tissue
Penis
Urethra
Rectum
Anus
Epididymis
Testis
Scrotum

MALE REPRODUCTIVE TRACT

1. The Scrotum and Testes

The scrotum is an organ that serves to contain the testes. Made out of skin and muscle, it is located in the pubic region, under the penis. It contains smooth muscles that allows it to contract and expand, thus keeping the testes closer or further to the body. This helps regulate their temperature, which has to be just right to support the spermatogenesis.

The testes, located within the scrotum, are responsible for production of sperm and the male hormone testosterone. The testes are connected to the abdomen by spermatic cords and cremaster muscles. The muscles serve to support the contraction and expansion of the scrotum.

On the inside, the testes are divided into small compartments, known as lobules, and these structures contain epithelial cells. In the epithelial cells, there are stem cells which form sperm cells. Wrapped around a portion of the testes, the epididymis is a coiled mass of tubes with combined lengths of several feet, in which the immature sperm matures before going further.

2. The Spermatic Ducts

The ductus deferens is muscular tube located within a spermatic cord, which carries the mature sperm from the epididymis, through the prostate, and to the ejaculatory tract. The ejaculatory tract is where the urethra and the ductus deferens meet. It also contains ducts from seminal vesicles.

The ejaculatory tract remains closed to the urethra until ejaculation, when it opens and expels the semen through the urethra. The urethra is a muscular tube located inside the penis. It serves both as a canal for expelling urine and semen.

3. **The Sex Glands**

Seminal vesicles, located between the urinary bladder and the rectum, are a pair of glands that produce the liquid part of the semen. The liquid contains proteins and has an alkaline pH, which allows the sperm to survive in the vagina's acidic environment. It also contains fructose, which serves as a source of energy for the sperm cells.

The prostate is a gland that surrounds the urethra and produces most of the liquid of the semen. It also contains smooth muscle which can constrict, to prevent the flow of semen or urine.

Cowper's glands are a pair of small glands located under the prostate. They secrete alkaline fluid that lubricates the urethra prior to ejaculation and removes the acidic remains of urine.

4. **The Penis**

The male sexual organ, the penis is the organ responsible for delivering the semen into the vagina. It is almost cylindrical in shape, and it contains the urethra and its external openings, as well as pockets of erectile tissue, which, when filled with blood, give the penis a larger size and stiffness.

The penis can be divided into three major regions:

- The root, which is where the penis is connected to the pelvis by ligaments.
- The body, which is the part that contains the most erectile tissue.
- The glans, the larger tip of the penis, is where the urethra ends and it also contains erectile tissue which makes it larger when filled with blood.

C. Physiology of the Reproductive System

The male reproductive system has only two functions: to produce the sperm and to fertilize the egg. The process of producing sperm is called spermatogenesis. It happens in the testes, and begins when males reach puberty, under the influence of hormones, including testosterone.

The fertilization is the process in which a sperm cell and an egg cell combine to form a fertilized zygote. After ejaculation, a sperm has to move through the vagina and uterus and get into the fallopian tube, where it comes in contact with an egg cell. If the sperm cell successfully penetrates the outer layer of the egg cell, their nuclei join and form a zygote, which then starts cellular division.

The female reproductive system produces the egg, plays its part in the fertilization, menstruates, carries the fetus, and feeds it after birth. Ovulation is the production process of a mature egg – the ovum. After fertilization, the zygote's cells develop rapidly and implant themselves into the wall of the urethra after about two weeks.

The endometrium, the lining of the vulva, prepares for a zygote while the ovum is traveling through the fallopian tube. If the fertilization does not happen, or the zygote does not implant itself successfully in the vulva, it cuts off the blood supply to the endometrium. This causes its cells to die off and the tissue to shred. This process is known as menstruation, and it happens each 28 days in regular, normal cycle.

If the fertilization is successful, and the zygote plants itself into the vulva, it will gradually grow from an embryo, into a fetus, and into a baby. The process of carrying and providing for the new life is called pregnancy. After the baby is born, the mother can breastfeed the child with the process called lactation, which is the production of the milk inside the breast's mammary glands.

Reproductive System Questions

1. The fallopian tubes connect:
   a) The vagina and the vulva
   b) The uterus and the vulva
   c) The ovaries and the uterus
   d) None of the Above

2. The ovaries are located:
   a) Inside the uterus
   b) On the left and right of the uterus
   c) On the top of the uterus
   d) None of the Above

3. Which of the following serves for exclusively for sexual pleasure?
   a) Clitoris
   b) Vagina
   c) Labia Minora
   d) None of the Above

4. Where are the mammary glands located?
   a) In the breast
   b) In the uterus
   c) Around the fallopian tubes
   d) None of the Above

5. Where are the testes located?
   a) Between the anus and the prostate
   b) In the scrotum
   c) Above the penis
   d) None of the Above

6. What is the role of the epididymis?
   a) It produces semen
   b) It keeps the temperature of the testes balanced
   c) It helps the sperm cells mature
   d) None of the Above

7. Which of the following produces the most fluid of the semen?
   a) The prostate
   b) The seminal vesicles
   c) The Cowper's glands
   d) None of the Above

8. The tip of the penis is called:
   a) The tip
   b) The head
   c) The glans
   d) None of the Above

The Reproductive System ANSWERS

1. C)
2. B)
3. A)
4. A)
5. B)
6. C)
7. A)
8. C)

Chapter 7: Physics

MOTION

Speed is a scalar quantity and is defined as distance divided by time. (Ex: miles per hour.)

Velocity is a vector quantity that describes speed and the direction of travel.

Magnitude of Acceleration is defined as the change in velocity divided by the time interval.

A **scalar quantity** is described only by its magnitude, whereas a **vector quantity** is described by magnitude and direction.

Acceleration is change in velocity divided by time; an object accelerates not only when it speeds up, but also when slowing down or turning. The **acceleration due to gravity** of a falling object near the Earth is a constant $9.8 m/s^2$; therefore an object's magnitude increases as it falls and decreases as it rises.

In most basic math, simple numerical values are calculated (for instance $1 + 1 = 2$). These simple numbers are known as **scalar** values, meaning they have a magnitude, but no direction, associated with them. Mass is an example of a scalar value commonly used in physics.

However, we live in a three-dimensional universe, so normally a simple number cannot sufficiently describe a physical characteristic. Instead, we need a magnitude as well as a direction, which is known as a **vector**. A vector not only tells how large a value is, but also whether it acts upward, to the left, to the right, etc.

For example, **speed** is a scalar value that tells you how fast an object is going. But if you are driving, knowing only the speed of your car, it will be impossible to navigate. Instead, you need to know your speed as well as the direction in which you are traveling, which is a vector value known as **velocity**. Velocity tells the direction and speed that an object is traveling.

Force and Newton's Laws of Motion

A **force** is a push or pull that can result in an object's motion or change of shape, and has a magnitude and direction, making it a vector. Force is measured in **Newtons** (N) in the metric system of units, but can also be measured in the standard unit of **pounds force** (lbf).

Though its effects can be noticed, a force cannot be seen; it can be thought of as an interaction between two bodies. The basic rules of forces are described by **Newton's Laws of Motion**, which are the foundation of the field of **mechanics.**

1. **First Law of Motion**: Until acted on by an external force, an object's velocity will remain constant, meaning speed and direction will not change. You may recognize: "An object at rest will remain at rest and an object in motion will remain in motion until a force is applied." An object's natural resistance to a change in its motion is known as **inertia**, so Newton's first law is also known as the **Law of Inertia**.

    Intuitively, the law of inertia makes sense. If a soccer ball is resting in a field, it is not going to move until someone kicks it. Once the ball is kicked, though, it does not continue to travel forever, which seems like it is a violation of Newton's first law.

However, there are forces such as drag from the air and friction from the field that eventually cause the ball to come to stop again. In the same way, if a moving car is put into neutral, it will slow down and eventually stop due to parasitic losses in the car's wheels and drivetrain, aero drag, and friction.

2. **Second Law of Motion**: Describes a force's effect on the motion of a body. It states that the acceleration of the object will be proportional to the sum of the forces being applied. Algebraically, Newton's second law is written as: $F = m * a$.

    Here, F is force, m is mass in kilograms (kg) or pounds mass (lbm), and a is acceleration in meters per second squared (m/s^2) or feet per second squared (ft/s^2). Notice that force and acceleration are both vectors, so the acceleration of an object will be in the direction of the force being applied to it.

    Acceleration is defined as the rate of change of an object's velocity. Acceleration does not have to result in a change in speed; it can also cause a change in direction, as is the case in centripetal, or rotational, acceleration. Remember that velocity and acceleration are two separate and distinct values. Just because the acceleration is positive does not mean that the object's velocity is positive and vice versa.

    A negative velocity would mean the object is going backward (or opposite of the direction designated as "positive") and a positive acceleration means the object's velocity is increasing in the positive direction (or decreasing in the negative direction). Though the term "deceleration" is often used to describe a decrease in speed, this is not technically correct. Instead, a change in velocity is always called acceleration and can either be positive or negative, depending on direction.

3. **Third Law of Motion**: Involves the coupling of forces and reactions. The law is often stated as, "For every action there is an equal and opposite reaction." The actions and reactions we are considering are forces. For example, if you lean against a wall, you are applying a force on the wall. According to Newton's third law, the wall is applying the same force back on you. These two forces will be the same magnitude, but in opposite directions; you push toward the wall and the wall pushes back on you. Because there is no motion involved when you lean again a wall, this is considered a **static** example.

    A **dynamic** example of Newton's third law is two cars crashing. If one car collides into a second, stationary car, both cars feel the same amount of force. The force applied to the stationary car is in the direction of the collision and causes the car to begin moving in the same direction as the first car. The moving car would have a force applied to it in the opposite direction by the stationary car, resulting in, among other things, a decrease in speed. Since the force on the two cars will be in opposite directions, the acceleration of the cars will also be in opposite directions; the stationary car speeds up and the moving car slows down.

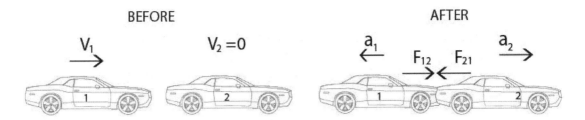

Collision of a car moving at velocity V_1 into the second stationary car with the force car 1 applies on car 2 F_1, the equal force car 2 applies on car 1 F_{21}, and the resulting accelerations a_1 and a_2.

There are **Three Important Conservation Laws** which are embodied within Newton's Laws. They offer a different and sometimes more powerful way to consider motion:

1. **Conservation of Momentum** – Embodied in Newton's first law (Law of Inertia), this reiterates that the momentum of a system is constant if no external forces act upon the system.

2. **Conservation of Energy** - Energy is neither created nor destroyed; it can be converted from one form to another (i.e. potential energy converted to kinetic energy), but the total amount of energy within the domain remains fixed.

3. **Conservation of Angular Momentum** – If the system is subjected to no external force, then the total angular momentum of a system has constant magnitude and direction. This is the common physics behind figure-skating and planetary orbits.

FRICTION

The normal force created by gravity also gives rise to a resistance to sliding known as **friction**. If you try to slide a refrigerator across a floor, you may find it very hard to move the object. Newton's third law suggests that there must be a force opposing your attempts to push the refrigerator; if not, it would easily slide across the floor and continue to slide until acted on by another force, such as a wall. This force opposing your efforts to move the refrigerator is friction. There are two types of friction: static and kinetic.

As you might have guessed, **static friction** is the force of friction between two objects that are not moving relative to each other. Static friction arises from the attempt to slide two surfaces past each other. In our refrigerator example, there is no force of friction until you attempt to push the refrigerator.

If you are not applying a force on the refrigerator, the only forces felt by the refrigerator are the force of gravity and the normal force of the floor holding it up, both of which are equal to the refrigerator's weight. When you start to push on the refrigerator and it does not move, static friction is holding the refrigerator in place.

The force of static friction is equal to the force that you are applying to the refrigerator; however, once pushed hard enough, the refrigerator will begin to move. The force necessary to start sliding an object is called **stiction** and is given by the equation: $F_{f,s} = \mu_s * N$.

$F_{f,s}$ is the maximum force of static friction (stiction), N is the normal force applied on the object by the surface across which it is sliding, and μ_s is the **coefficient of static friction**. Past this stiction point, the object will begin to move, and the force of **kinetic friction** will oppose the sliding motion: $F_{f,k} = \mu_k * N$. This is the same as the equation for static friction, except that the coefficient μ_k is the **coefficient of kinetic friction**.

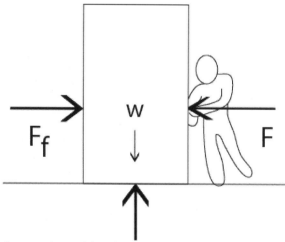

The force of friction, whether static or kinetic, will always oppose the direction of the force causing the sliding. Also, both coefficients of friction are always less than one, and the coefficient of static friction is usually greater than the coefficient of kinetic friction.

This means that it takes a greater force to get an object to start sliding across a surface than it does to keep the object sliding once it has already started. The figure following [LL4]shows a graph of the force of friction versus the sliding force applied to an object.

Considering this graph in relation to our refrigerator example, if you start pushing on the refrigerator, the force of static friction will prevent sliding until you have applied enough force to overcome the stiction point. After this, the force of kinetic friction will give a constant opposition to the sliding, no matter how hard or fast you push.

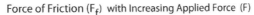

Force of Friction (F_f) with Increasing Applied Force (F)

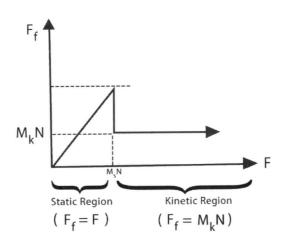

ENERGY

An object raised to a height above the ground will have an amount of stored energy known as **gravitational potential energy**. The higher an object is moved, the more potential it has. Gravitational potential energy is defined as: $PE = m * g * h$.

Here, m is the mass of the object, g is the acceleration of gravity (9.81 m/s^2), and h is the height of the object from the surface of the earth.

Sometimes, gravitational potential energy is represented by the letter U instead of PE.

Gravitational potential energy, like all types of energy, is given in units of joules (J) or foot-pounds-force (ft-lbf). You may notice that gravitational potential energy is simply the force of gravity on an object multiplied by the objects height.

Since the force of gravity, or weight, is given in units of Newtons, one joule is the same as one Newton multiplied by one meter (1J = 1Nm). When an object is dropped, its gravitational potential energy is converted into **kinetic energy**, which is defined as: $KE = \frac{1}{2} m * v^2$.

Here, m is again the mass of the object and v is the object's velocity.

Kinetic energy also has units of joules and is sometimes represented by the letter E instead of KE. Energy is always conserved, meaning it cannot be created or destroyed. This is known as the law of **conservation of energy**. The law of conservation of gravitational energy can be written as:
$PE + KE = m * g * h + \frac{1}{2} m * v^2 = $ constant.

However, all types of energy are always conserved, whether mechanical, electrical, chemical, nuclear, solar, etc. Even the power plants that supply our homes with electricity do not create energy; they simply convert kinetic, chemical, nuclear, or solar energy into electrical energy.

If an object is brought to a certain height, it has a particular amount of gravitational potential energy. When the object is dropped, its potential energy is converted to kinetic energy, so the amount of gravitational potential energy that the object had at its highest point will be exactly how much kinetic energy it has as it hits the ground (ignoring aero drag).

The law of conservation of energy applies to all objects in a gravitational field, so the velocity of a falling object will depend only on the height through which it has fallen and not the path. This means that the same laws used to find the speed of a falling baseball can also be used to find the speed of a rollercoaster.

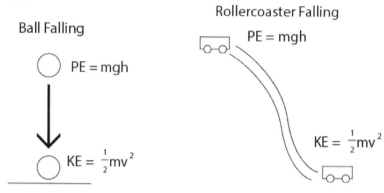

THERMAL PHYSICS
Temperature and Heat
Heat and temperature are two different things. **Heat** is a measure of the work required to change the speeds in a collection of atoms or molecules. **Temperature** is a measure of the average kinetic energy of the atoms or molecules of a substance.

A **calorie** is the amount of heat required to raise the temperature of 1 gram of water by 1 degree Celsius. The **specific heat** of a substance is the ratio of the amount of heat added to a substance, divided by the mass and the temperature change of the substance.

The change of a substance from solid to liquid, or liquid to gas, etc., is called a **phase change**.

> **Heat of Fusion:** The amount of heat required to change a unit mass of a substance from solid to liquid at the *melting point*.

> **Heat of Vaporization:** The amount of heat needed to change a unit mass of a substance from liquid to vapor at the *boiling point*.

HEAT TRANSFER
Temperature Scales
There are three common temperature scales: **Celsius**, **Fahrenheit**, and **Kelvin**. Because it is based upon what we believe to be **absolute zero** (the lowest theoretical temperature possible before life ceases), the Kelvin scale is also known as the **absolute scale**.

Temperature Scale	Point at Which Water Freezes
Celsius	0° C
Fahrenheit	32° F
Kelvin	273K

The Two Mechanisms of Heat Transfer

Conduction: Heat transfer via conduction can occur in a substance of any phase (solid, liquid, or gas), but is mostly seen in solids.

Convection: Convection heat transfer occurs only in fluids (liquids and gases).

Both types of heat transfer are caused by molecular movement in the substance of interest.

WAVE MOTION (SOUND) AND MAGNETISM
Waves
Waves can be placed in one of two categories: **longitudinal** or **transverse**.

In a **transverse wave**, the motion of the medium is perpendicular to the motion of the wave; for example, waves on water. In a **longitudinal wave**, the motion of the medium is parallel to the motion of the wave. Sound waves are transverse waves.

A wave's **wavelength** is the distance between successive high points (**crests**) and low points (**troughs**). The **speed of a wave** is the rate at which it moves. **Frequency** – measured in **Hertz** (Hz) – is the number of repetitions, or cycles, occurring per second. The **amplitude** is the intensity (or strength) of the wave.

Sound
When vibrations disturb the air, they create sound waves. The **speed of a sound wave** is approximately 331m/s at 0° C. Human ears are capable of hearing frequencies between 20 to 16,000 Hz. The **decibel** (dB) scale is used to measure the loudness (amount of energy) of a sound wave. The scale starts at zero, which is the softest audio, and increases tenfold in intensity for every 10dB.

NATURE OF ELECTRICITY

Magnetism is a force which either pulls magnetic materials together or pushes them apart. Iron and nickel are the most common magnetic materials. All magnetic materials are made up of tiny groups of atoms called domains. Each domain is like a mini-magnet with north and south poles. When material is magnetized, millions of domains line up.

Around every magnet there is a region in which its effects are felt, called its **magnetic field**. The magnetic field around a planet or a star is called the **magnetosphere**. Most of the planets in the Solar System, including Earth, have a magnetic field. Planets have magnetic fields because of the liquid iron in their cores. As the planets rotate, so does the iron swirl, generating electric currents which create a magnetic field. The strength of a magnet is measured in **teslas**. The Earth's magnetic field is 0.00005 teslas.

An electric current creates its own magnetic field. **Electromagnetism** (the force created together by magnetism and electricity) is one of the four fundamental forces in the Universe; the other three are gravity and the two basic forces of the atomic nucleus.

A magnet has two poles: a north pole and a south pole. Like (similar) poles (e.g. two north poles) repel each other; unlike poles attract each other. The Earth has a magnetic field that is created by electric currents within its iron core. The magnetic north pole is close to the geographic North Pole. If left to swivel freely, a magnet will turn so that its north pole points to the Earth's magnetic north pole.

In the modern world, electronics are all around us and we each rely on electricity for our basic needs. Despite its presence in all aspects of our lives, electricity is not often fully understood. However, as electronics become more and more prevalent in everyday life, it is becoming increasingly important for one to have a basic knowledge of electricity.

Atoms and the Electrical Current

Many find the concept of electricity difficult to comprehend because electricity cannot be seen. This is because electricity originates at the subatomic level. All objects are made of **atoms**, including this book, the chair you are sitting in, and even you.

Atoms are made of protons, neutrons, and electrons. Protons and neutrons make up the **nucleus** of an atom, and electrons orbit around the nucleus in layers known as **shells**.

Protons: Positively charged particles.

Electrons: Negatively charged particles.

Neutrons: Particles without charge.

Let's have an example.

The picture below shows the basic structure of an aluminum atom. Aluminum's atomic number is 13, as seen on a periodic table of elements. This **atomic number** tells the total number of electrons in a single atom. To balance the negative charge of the electrons, an atom has the same number of protons as electrons, so the aluminum atom in the figure has 13 protons in its nucleus.

Aluminum's Atomic Structure

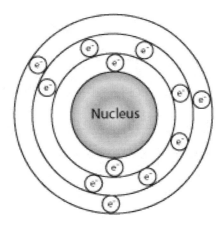

Also note that the aluminum atom only has three electrons in its outer shell. This outer shell, known as the **valence shell**, is what determines the conductivity of an object. **Conductivity** refers to the willingness of atoms to exchange electrons. Aluminum is highly conductive because its outer shell is capable of holding eight electrons, like the noble gas argon, but a single atom only has three electrons in its valence shell. This means it has a tendency to steal or share electrons through ionic and covalent bonds when it is combined with other atoms.

Materials can be divided into three broad categories: **conductors**, **insulators**, and **semi-conductors**.

Conductors
When the atoms of a material easily exchange electrons, the material is said to be a **conductor**.

Valence electrons in conductors have low ionization energy, which means that it does not take as much energy to separate valence electrons from the atom. This is because the valence shell is not filled, which allows the valence electrons to easily move to a neighboring atom.

As we will find later, it is this movement of electrons that gives rise to electricity. Metals are good conductors in their solid state and often have **free electrons** that do not belong to a single atom but move freely throughout the material's volume. Silver, copper, and gold are the most conductive metals. While silver is more conductive than copper, it is also more expensive, which is why it is common to see copper used in household items.

Insulators
Atoms in **insulators** do not easily exchange electrons. The ionization energy of these elements is much greater than conductors because the valence shells are filled (or the electrons present in the outer shell are bonding with neighboring atoms).

Rubbers, plastics, and ceramics are categorized as insulators, which is why these are also often seen in home appliances, such as plastic insulation around metal wires, ceramic circuit boards, and PVC conduit.

Semi-conductors

Semi-conductors behave as neither conductors nor insulators. However, they can have very interesting uses that will be discussed in detail later.

As was stated earlier, the flow of electrons gives rise to electricity. However, we have not yet mentioned what makes these electrons move from one atom to another. The answer is an **electrical potential** difference, or change in **voltage**, across the material, usually provided by a battery or power source.

A battery has two terminals: one positive and one negative. The negative terminal has a negative charge because it has an excess of electrons relative to the positive terminal (remember that electrons are negatively charged).

When a wire is used to connect the two terminals, there is a voltage difference across the wire that creates an electric field within the wire. This begins to push electrons toward the positive terminal in an attempt to neutralize the voltage difference.

This is similar to a situation in which two tanks, one full and one empty, are connected by a pipe near the base. If the pipe is opened, the water will flow from the full tank into the empty tank until the levels are equal.

This is why electrical potential, or the ability to accomplish electrical work, is also called **electrical pressure**; it is the driving force of electricity through a conductor, just as pressure is the driving force of water through a pipe.

Electrical potential is also known as **electromotive force** (emf) because it can be thought of as the force that causes electrons to move through a conductor. In equations, electrical potential is represented with the letter E. Electrical potential is measured as voltage in units called **volts** (V). To measure voltage, a **voltmeter** is connected to the two points of the circuit across which the voltage drop is being found.

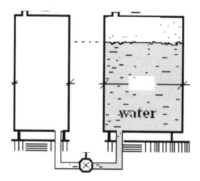

Think again about the wire connected to a battery's terminals; a certain number of electrons will flow past a given point each second, and each of these electrons carries a certain **charge** (Approximately $-1.602 * 10^{-19}$ Coulombs).

The flow rate of electrical charge is called **current**, which can be measured by attaching an **ammeter** into a circuit at the point through which it is desired to measure current. Current is measured in amperes (A), or **amps**, and one amp is equal to one coulomb per second. In formulae, current is represented by the letter I, which can be remembered by thinking of current as the *intensity* of electrical flow.

Current is the flow rate of electrical charge, but electrons are negatively charged. This means that current is not given by the direction of the flow of electrons, but opposes the flow of electrons. While electrons flow from lower to higher electric potential, electricity flows from high to low electric potential. This convention can be confusing, but the thing to remember is that electrons flow in order to equalize electric potential and, because electrons are negative, current flows in the opposite direction.

240

In our battery example, excess electrons flow from the negative terminal towards the positive, and because the electrons have a negative charge, the charge is actually said to be flowing from the positive terminal toward the negative terminal. Thus electrical current can always be thought of as opposing the flow of electrons.

So far in our discussion of electricity, we have only considered the battery as a power source. In this example, we are provided with a relatively constant voltage, so the current flowing through our wire will be constant as well. This flow of current in a single direction is known as **direct current** (DC) and can be seen in cars and other battery-powered appliances as well as thermocouples and solar cells.

The electricity provided by the outlets in our houses, however, is known as **alternating current** (AC) and does not flow in a single direction. Instead, the voltage oscillates, changing directions to back and forth very quickly, usually creating a smooth sine-wave when graphed against time (See figure on the next page). [LL5]

The advantage to supplying this AC power to residents and businesses is that it can be transmitted through great distances at high voltages; transformers can be used to either increase or decrease the voltage. AC does not always create a nice sine-wave when graphed, though. In some applications, it will create a square or triangular wave or any other shape imaginable.

In laboratories, an instrument called an oscilloscope is used to create various AC wave patterns, such as the ones shown in the graphs below, with a given frequency and wavelength. **Frequency** is measured in units of hertz (Hz), which is the number of complete cycles per second. **Wavelength** is the distance between two consecutive peaks or troughs in a wave. The waves shown below [LL6]all have the same wavelength and frequency.

In America, electricity is provided at 120 V and 60 Hz. This means that in America the current from our outlets changes directions a total of 120 times, creating 60 full waves, every second. Often home appliances will have an AC/DC adapter, known as a recifier. Other countries do not necessarily provide electricity at the same voltage and frequency, so it is important not to attempt to use American appliances outside of the country without knowing the type of power being supplied and using the appropriate adapter.

Figure 1.4: Wave created by alternating current

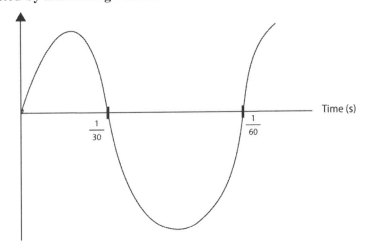

Figure 1.5: Common AC Wave Patterns

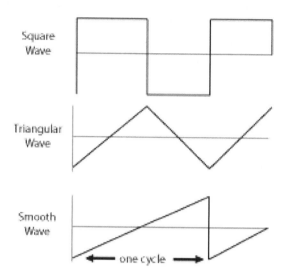

Circuits and Diagrams

A **circuit** is a chain of electrical components that includes a power source, conductors, and loads. A **closed-loop**, meaning a continuous path connecting the positive and negative ends of a power supply, is necessary for the flow of electricity to be possible. We have considered a circuit with a battery and a wire conductor. [ER7]This circuit accomplishes nothing besides draining our battery and creating heat in the wire. Usually an electrical circuit is designed to convert electrical energy into some other useable form of energy such as movement or light.

CENTRIFUGAL FORCE

The terms centripetal and centrifugal force are often incorrectly used interchangeably. A **centripetal force** is a force that makes an object travel along a curved path. This means a centripetal force creates a **centripetal acceleration** toward the center of the curved path.

For example, when a car is driven in a circle, the front tires exert a centripetal force on the car, accelerating it toward the center of the circle. Passengers in the car feel as though they are being pulled toward the outside of the circle, and this pull is **centrifugal acceleration**, which results from **centrifugal force**.

A centrifugal force is the reaction force of a centripetal force that pulls an object toward the outside of the curved path being traveled. This all means that a centrifugal force and a centripetal force are of equal magnitude and opposite directions, just as would be expected of a force and reaction according to Newton's third law. As Newton's second law states, centripetal force equals the mass of the object multiplied by centripetal acceleration:

$$F_c = m * a_c = m * v^2/R$$

Here, a_c is the centripetal acceleration and is equal to the square of the object's linear velocity (v) divided by the radius of the curved path, R.

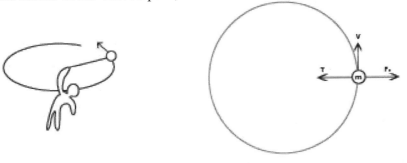

When a ball on a string is swung in a circle, the string exerts a centripetal force on the ball, preventing it from leaving the circular path, and the resulting centrifugal force pulls the ball outward, causing tension in the string and keeping it taut.

243

Test Your Knowledge: Physics

1. The temperature at which all molecular motion stops is:
   a) −460 °C.
   b) −273 K.
   c) 0 K.
   d) 0C.

2. _____is the amount of heat required to raise the temperature of 1 gram of water by 1 degree Celsius.
   a) Specific heat
   b) Heat of fusion
   c) calorie
   d) Heat of vaporization

3. An object that has kinetic energy must be:
   a) Moving.
   b) Falling.
   c) At an elevated position.
   d) At rest.

4. The amount of heat required to melt an ice cube is called:
   a) Conduction.
   b) Specific Heat.
   c) A calorie.
   d) Heat of fusion.

5. A moving object has
   a) Velocity.
   b) Momentum.
   c) Energy.
   d) All of these.

6. Heat transferred between a pot of boiling water and the air above it is an example of:
   a) Conduction.
   b) Convection.
   c) Heat of vaporization.
   d) Phase change.

7. _____ increases, decreases, or changes the direction of a force is:
   a) A simple machine.
   b) Energy.
   c) Momentum.
   d) Inertia.

8. _____ is a measure of the average kinetic energy of the atoms or molecules of a substance.
   a) Specific Heat
   b) Temperature
   c) Heat
   d) Force

9. Average speed is:
   a) A measure of how fast something is moving.
   b) The distance covered per unit of time.
   c) Always measured in terms of a unit of distance divided by a unit of time.
   d) All of the above.

10. Which of the following controls can change a car's velocity?
   a) The steering wheel.
   b) The brake pedal.
   c) Both A and B.
   d) None of the above.

11. The distance between two corresponding parts of a wave.
   a) Wavelength.
   b) Crest.
   c) Energy.
   d) Equidistance.

12. The high part of a transverse wave.
   a) Height.
   b) Period.
   c) Crest.
   d) Wavelength.

13. The magnetic field around a planet or a star is called a(an):
   a) Electromagnetic field.
   b) Magnetosphere.
   c) Magnetic field.
   d) Magnetic energy field.

14. The number of waves that pass a given point in one second.
- a) Trough.
- b) Energy.
- c) Crest.
- d) Frequency.

Test Your Knowledge: Physics – Answers

1. **c)**

2. **c)**

3. **a)**

4. **d)**

5. **d)**

6. **b)**

7. **a)**

8. **b)**

9. **d)**

10. **c)**

11. **a)**

12. **c)**

13. **b)**

14. **d)**

HESI A2 PRACTICE TEST #1

Mathematics Practice Test #1

1. $(5 * 3) * 1 + 5 =$

2. $(7^2 - 2^3 - 6) =$

3. $(5^3 + 7) * 2 =$

4. $0.98 + 45.102 + 32.3333 + 31 + 0.00009 =$
   a) 368.573
   b) 210.536299
   c) 109.41539
   d) 99.9975

5. $0.12 \div 1 =$
   a) 12
   b) 1.2
   c) .12
   d) .012

6. $(9 \div 3) * (8 \div 4) =$
   a) 1
   b) 6
   c) 72
   d) 576

7. $6 * 0 * 5 =$
   a) 30
   b) 11
   c) 25
   d) 0

8. $7.95 \div 1.5 =$
   a) 2.4
   b) 5.3
   c) 6.2
   d) 7.3

9. A basket has 36 apples and oranges, with 12 more apples than oranges. How many apples are there?
   a) 12
   b) 15
   c) 24
   d) 28

10. What is the next number in the sequence? 6, 12, 24, 48, ___.

    a) 72

    b) 96

    c) 108

    d) 112

11. If the perimeter of a rectangular house is 44 yards, and the length is 36 feet, what is its width?

    a) 30 feet.

    b) 18 yards.

    c) 28 feet.

    d) 32 feet.

12. If a discount of 25% off the retail price of a desk saves Mark $45, what was the desk's original price?

    a) $135

    b) $160

    c) $180

    d) $210

13. Joey pays $1,100 in taxes on his car. What is the value of the car, if taxes are 8.9% of the value?

    a) $9,765.45.

    b) $10,876.90.

    c) $12,359.55.

    d) $14,345.48.

14. How many years does Steven need to invest his $3,000 at 7% to earn $210 in simple interest?

    a) 1 year.

    b) 2 years.

    c) 3 years.

    d) 4 years.

15. 35% of what number is 70?

    a) 100

    b) 110

    c) 150

    d) 200

16. What number is 5% of 2000?

    a) 50

    b) 100

    c) 150

    d) 200

17. 9.86 + 1.27 =
- a) 11.13
- b) 13.13
- c) 11.11
- d) 10.13

18. 5 + 11.75 + 7.22 =
- a) 25.76
- b) 22.91
- c) 23.97
- d) 23.47

19. 15.15 + 1.51 =
- a) 16.52
- b) 17.66
- c) 15.76
- d) 16.66

20. 27.23 + 5.65 =
- a) 32.88
- b) 33.56
- c) 32.25
- d) 33.65

21. 18.25 + 1.17 + 5.24 =
- a) 23.56
- b) 24.66
- c) 25.66
- d) 24.36

22. 22.22 – 11.11 =
- a) 11.22
- b) 10.11
- c) 11.11
- d) 10.10

23. 4.22 – 1.37 =
- a) 2.85
- b) 3.85
- c) 2.58
- d) 2.35

24. 11.7 – 4.8 =
- a) 6.61
- b) 6.50
- c) 7.90
- d) 6.90

25. 5.82 – 2.17 =
- a) 3.46
- b) 3.65
- c) 4.65
- d) 3.25

26. 16.8 – 7.4 =
- a) 9.6
- b) 8.4
- c) 9.2
- d) 9.4

27. 99 * 0.45 =
- a) 45.50
- b) 55.45
- c) 44.55
- d) 45.55

28. 7.5 * 3 =
- a) 21.25
- b) 22.50
- c) 23
- d) 23.50

29. How many milligrams are in a gram?
- a) 10
- b) 100
- c) 500
- d) 1,000

30. How many pounds are in a kilogram?
- a) 2.2
- b) 4.85
- c) 0.45
- d) 0.22

31. How many meters in one kilometer?
- a) 10.
- b) 100.
- c) 1,000.
- d) 10,000.

32. How many centimeters in one meter?
   a) 10
   b) 100
   c) 1,000
   d) 10,000

33. If a shift is 1500 to 2300 hours, what time does the shift start?
   a) 1:50 am.
   b) 2:00 pm.
   c) 3:00 pm.
   d) 11:00 am.

34. How is 7:45 pm, expressed in military time?
   a) 1545
   b) 1745
   c) 0745
   d) 1945

35. $\frac{2}{8} + \frac{3}{8} =$

   a) $\frac{5}{8}$

   b) $\frac{5}{49}$

   c) $\frac{5}{64}$

   d) $\frac{5}{16}$

36. $\frac{3}{5} \div \frac{1}{10} =$

   a) 3
   b) 3/5
   c) 6
   d) 2.5

37. $\dfrac{2}{7} * \dfrac{3}{7} =$

    a) $\dfrac{5}{7}$

    b) $\dfrac{6}{49}$

    c) $\dfrac{7}{42}$

    d) $\dfrac{5}{14}$

38. What is decimal form of 5/45?
    a. 0.23
    b. 0.7
    c. 0.55
    d. 0.11

39. What is the decimal form of 7/8?
    a. 0.875
    b. 0.755
    c. 0.625
    d. 0.450

40. What is the decimal form of 3/15?
    a. 0.3
    b. 0.2
    c. 0.25
    d. 0.4

41. What is the decimal form of 9/20?
    a. 0.3
    b. 0.35
    c. 0.4
    d. 0.45

42. Convert 0.95 to a fraction.
    a. 15/20
    b. 19/20
    c. 7/9
    d. 14/25

43. Convert .625 to a fraction.

     a. 4/7

     b. 3/8

     c. 5/8

     d. 3/10

44. Convert 0.700 to a fraction

     a. 5/9

     b. 7/10

     c. 7/9

     d. 3/8

45. If Lynn can type a page in p minutes, how many pages can she do in 5 minutes?

     a) $5/p$.

     b) $p - 5$.

     c) $p + 5$.

     d) $p/5$.

46. A computer is on sale for $1,600, which is a 20% discount off the regular price. The regular price is?

     a) $1800.

     b) $1900.

     c) $2000.

     d) $2100.

47. The city council has decided to add a 0.3% tax on motel and hotel rooms. If a traveler spends the night in a motel room that costs $55 before taxes, how much will the city receive in taxes from him?

     a) 10 cents.

     b) 11 cents.

     c) 15 cents.

     d) 17 cents.

48. You need to purchase a textbook for nursing school. The book costs $80.00, and the sales tax is 8.25%. You have $100. How much change will you receive back?

    a) $5.20.
    b) $7.35.
    c) $13.40.
    d) $19.95.

49. Jim's belt broke, and his pants are falling down. He has 5 pieces of string. He needs to choose the piece that will be able to go around his 36-inch waist. The piece must be at least 4 inches longer than his waist so that he can tie a knot in it, but it cannot be more that 6 inches longer so that the ends will not show from under his shirt. Which of the following pieces of string will work the best?

    a) 3 feet.
    b) 3 ¾ feet.
    c) 3 5/8 feet.
    d) 3 1/3 feet.

50. During a 5-day festival, the number of visitors tripled each day. If the festival opened on a Thursday with 345 visitors, what was the attendance on that Sunday?

    a) 345.
    b) 1,035.
    c) 1,725.
    d) 9,315.

HESI A2 Mathematics Practice Test #1 – Answers

1. **Answer: 20**
   Explanation: This question also involves the order of operations (PEMDAS). To solve this question, we solve the parenthesis first, and then multiply the answer by 1. After that, we add 5 to get our final answer. (5*3) = 15, so the expression becomes 15*1+5 = 15 + 5 = 20

2. **Answer: 35**
   Explanation: We need to remember the order of operations (PEMDAS) to solve this question. First of all, we solve the parenthesis, and then the exponents. However, in order to solve the parenthesis, we need to know the values of 7^2 and 2^3. Therefore, we find these exponents first and then proceed with PEMDAS. Since $7^2 = 49$ and $2^3 = 8$, the expression becomes (49-8-6) i.e. we simply subtract 6 and 8 from 49 to get our final answer which is equal to 35.

3. **Answer: 264**
   Explanation: First of all, we find the value of 5^3 to solve the parenthesis (remember the order of operations PEMDAS). As we know that $5^3 = 5*5*5 = 125$, the expression becomes (125+7)*2.
   We solve the parenthesis first because it is given more preference in PEMDAS, it becomes132*2.
   Multiplying these two numbers, we get our final answer which is 264.

4. **Answer choice: c) 109.41539**

5. **Answer choice c) 0.12**

6. **Answer choice b) 72**

7. **Answer choice d) 0**

8. **Answer choice b) 5.3**

9. **Answer choice c) 24**

10. **Answer choice b) 96**

11. **Answer choice a) 30 Feet**

12. **Answer choice c) $180**

13. **Answer choice c) $12,349.55**

14. **Answer choice a) 1 year**

15. **Answer choice d) 200**

16. **Answer choice b) 100**

17. **Answer choice a) 11.13**

18. **Answer choice c) 23.97**

19. **Answer choice d) 16.66**

20. Answer choice a) 32.88

21. Answer choice b) 24.66

22. Answer choice c) 11.11

23. Answer choice a) 2.85

24. Answer choice d) 6.90

25. Answer choice b) 3.65

26. Answer choice d) 9.4

27. Answer choice c) 44.55

28. Answer choice b) 22.50

29. Answer choice d) 1,000

30. Answer choice a) 2.2 pounds/kilo

31. Answer choice c) 1,000

32. Answer choice b) 100

33. Answer choice c) 3:00pm

34. Answer choice d) 1945

35. Answer choice a) $\frac{5}{8}$

36. Answer choice c) 6

37. Answer choice b) $\frac{6}{49}$

38. Answer choice d) 0.11

39. Answer choice a) 0.875

40. Answer choice b) 0.2

41. Answer choice d) 0.45

42. Answer choice b) 19/20

43. Answer choice c) 5/8

44. Answer choice b) 7/10

45. a) Explanation: From the given information in the question, Lynn writes one page in 'p' minutes. Now, we are asked about the number of pages Lynn can write in 5 minutes. The simplest way to solve this question is by writing it in ratio form I.e.

1 page ➜ 'p' minutes

X pages ➜ 5 minutes

Cross multiplying the above equations, we get 5*1 =x*p

Therefore, x = 5/p (Which means that he can type 5/p pages in 5 minutes)

46. c) Explanation: From the statement of the question, it is clear that when we take 20% off the price of computer, it costs $1600. This means that $1600 equals 80% of the actual price of the computer. Writing this in form of an equation;

0.8 * x = $1600

x = 1600/0.8

x = $2000 where 'x' is the actual price of the computer.

47. d)Explanation: Hotel chares a tax of 0.3% i.e. 0.3/100 = 0.003. Multiplying it with $55 gives us the amount of tax amount which hotel has charged to this traveler.

$55* 0.003 = $0.165

Note that the given answer choices are in cents and our answer is in dollars. We convert our answer in to cents by multiplying it with 100. It becomes 16.5 cents. The nearest possible option 17 cents which is Option (d).

48. c) Explanation: This is a tricky question. We are given with the sales tax percentage and the actual amount of the book. First of all, we need to find out the amount we would be charged for this including sales tax, and then we need to subtract it from 100, to find out   the   change   we   will   receive   from   them. 8.5% tax on $80 becomes 0.085*80 = $6.8

So, the total amount that we will be charged becomes 80+ 6.8 = $86.8

Subtracting it from $100 to find the change, we get 100 – 86.8 = $13.40

49. d) Explanation: From the statement of the question, it is clear that we need string that is at least 40 inches long (i.e. 36 inch waist and 4 inches for knot) but not longer than 42 inches.

Let's examine the length of strings available in answer options.

Option (a) = 3 feet = 36 inches Incorrect

Option (b) = 3(3/4) feet = 45 inches Incorrect

Option (c) = 3(5/8) feet = 43.5 inches Incorrect

Option (d) = 3 (1/3) feet = 40 inches **Correct**

Option (e) = 2(1/2) feet = 30 inches Incorrect

50. d) Explanation: The number of people on Thursday is 345. Every next day the number of people triples. On Friday, it becomes 3*345 = 1035

On Saturday, the number of people who came to this festival became 3 * 1035 =3105

On Sunday, the number of people who came to this festival became 3 * 3105 = 9315

Reading Section Practice Test #1

Many persons plead a love of truth as an apology for rough manners, as if truth was never gentle and kind, but always harsh, morose, and forbidding. Surely good manners and a good conscience are no more inconsistent with each other than beauty and innocence, which are strikingly akin, and always look the better for companionship. Roughness and honesty are indeed sometimes found together in the same person, but he is a poor judge of human nature who takes ill-manners to be a guarantee of probity of character. Some persons object to politeness, that its language is unmeaning and false. But this is easily answered. A lie is not locked up in a phrase, but must exist, if at all, in the mind of the speaker. In the ordinary compliments of civilized life, there is no intention to deceive, and consequently no falsehood. Polite language is pleasant to the ear, and soothing to the heart, while rough words are just the reverse; and if not the product of ill temper, are very apt to produce it. The plainest of truths, let it be remembered, can be conveyed in civil speech, while the most malignant lies may find utterance, and often do, in the language of the fish market.

1. What is the main idea of the passage?
    a. Fishmongers have bad manners.
    b. Good manners and honesty can go together.
    c. A little white lie is necessary for politeness.
    d. Poor manners are not a sign of honesty.

2. Which statement is not a detail from the passage?
    a. Truth can be gentle and kind.
    b. Honesty is often an excuse for bad manners.
    c. Lies can be conveyed with rough manners.
    d. People with good manners intend to deceive.

3. What is the meaning of <u>deceive</u> near the end of the paragraph?
    a. Make someone believe something that is not true
    b. Convince someone to give you something
    c. Spread an unkind story about someone else
    d. Share truths or speak honestly

4. What is the author's primary purpose in writing this passage?
    a. To emphasize the importance of honesty
    b. To share information about fish markets
    c. To talk about the differences in manners among the social classes
    d. To explain that manners and honesty can coexist

5. Which is the best summary of this passage?
    a. Civil speech helps people to get along.
    b. Honesty is always the best policy.
    c. Good manners help you to lie.
    d. Rough manners cause fights.

"However, let us go to dinner, and I will soon tell you whether you are a well-bred man or not; and here let me premise that what is good manners for a small dinner is good manners for a large one, and vice versâ. Now, the first thing you do is to sit down. Stop, sir! Pray do not cram yourself into the table in that way; no, nor sit a yard from it, like that. How graceless, inconvenient, and in the way of conversation! Why, dear me! You are positively putting your elbows on the table, and now you have got your hands fumbling about with the spoons and forks, and now you are nearly knocking my new hock glasses over. Can't you take your hands down, sir? Didn't you learn that in the nursery? Didn't your mamma say to you, 'Never put your hands above the table except to carve or eat?' Oh! But come, no nonsense, sit up, if you please. I can't have your fine head of hair forming a side dish on my table; you must not bury your face in the plate, you came to show it, and it ought to be alive. Well, but there is no occasion to throw your head back like that, you look like an alderman, sir, after dinner. Pray, don't lounge in that sleepy way. You are here to eat, drink, and be merry. You can sleep when you get home.

6. What is the main idea of the passage?
   a. Aldermen drink too much.
   b. Well-bred individuals have good manners.
   c. You should not nap at the dinner table.
   d. Don't put your hands above the table.

7. Which statement is not a detail from the passage?
   a. Don't put your hands above the table.
   b. Don't sit a yard from the table.
   c. Don't lean over your plate.
   d. Don't put your elbows on the table.

8. What is the meaning of <u>lounge</u> near the end of the paragraph?
   a. Couch or sofa
   b. Lay down
   c. Sleep
   d. Relax

9. What is the author's primary purpose in writing this passage?
   a. To teach manners.
   b. To amuse the reader.
   c. To explain why you should not go to dinner parties.
   d. To illustrate how to properly eat fish.

10. Which is the best summary of this passage?
   a. Good manners are common sense.
   b. Use good manners at meals.
   c. No one has good manners.
   d. Good manners are unimportant

I do not mean to prescribe rules to strong and valiant natures, who will mind their own affairs whether in heaven or hell, and perchance build more magnificently and spend more lavishly than the richest, without ever impoverishing themselves, not knowing how they live—if, indeed, there are any such, as has been dreamed; nor to those who find their encouragement and inspiration in precisely the present condition of things, and cherish it with the fondness and enthusiasm of lovers—and, to some extent, I reckon myself in this number; I do not speak to those who are well employed, in whatever circumstances, and they know whether they are well employed or not;—but mainly to the mass of men who are discontented, and idly complaining of the hardness of their lot or of the times, when they might improve them. There are some who complain most energetically and inconsolably of any, because they are, as they say, doing their duty. I also have in my mind that seemingly wealthy, but most terribly impoverished class of all, who have accumulated dross, but know not how to use it, or get rid of it, and thus have forged their own golden or silver fetters.

11. What is the main idea of the passage?
    a. Spending money will provide happiness.
    b. Poverty will cause unhappiness.
    c. Money does not necessarily provide happiness.
    d. Happiness requires wealth.

12. Which statement is not a detail from the passage?
    a. The author is discontent.
    b. The author is happy with his life.
    c. The wealthy can be happy.
    d. The wealthy can be unhappy.

13. What is the meaning of <u>discontented</u> in the paragraph?
    a. Happy
    b. Unhappy
    c. Rich
    d. Poor

14. What is the author's primary purpose in writing this passage?
    a. The author is identifying his reader.
    b. The author is praising the reader.
    c. The author is criticizing the reader.
    d. The author is distancing himself from the reader.

15. Which is the best summary of this passage?
    a. Money can buy happiness.
    b. Wealth cannot buy happiness.
    c. If you are rich, you cannot be happy.
    d. Happiness requires more than wealth.

The world is very different now. For man holds in his mortal hands the power to abolish all forms of human poverty and all forms of human life. And yet the same revolutionary beliefs for which our forebears fought are still at issue around the globe--the belief that the rights of man come not from the generosity of the state, but from the hand of God.

We dare not forget today that we are the heirs of that first revolution. Let the word go forth from this time and place, to friend and foe alike, that the torch has been passed to a new generation of Americans--born in this century, tempered by war, disciplined by a hard and bitter peace, proud of our ancient heritage, and unwilling to witness or permit the slow undoing of those human rights to which this nation has always been committed, and to which we are committed today at home and around the world.

Let every nation know, whether it wishes us well or ill, that we shall pay any price, bear any burden, meet any hardship, support any friend, oppose any foe, to assure the survival and the success of liberty.

16. What is the main idea of the passage?
    a. Americans will not fight for freedom.
    b. Americans are concerned with internal issues.
    c. Americans will support freedom around the world.
    d. Americans have recently fought a war.

17. Which statement is not a detail from the passage?
    a. World War II caused many deaths.
    b. Americans are committed to human rights.
    c. America will accept losses to support freedom.
    d. Freedom does not come from the generosity of the state.

18. What is the meaning of abolish in the first paragraph?
    a. To start something
    b. To bring an end to something
    c. To commit to something
    d. To condemn something

19. What is the author's primary purpose in writing this passage?
    a. To condemn war
    b. To support peace
    c. To inspire others
    d. To educate

20. Which is the best summary of this passage?
    a. Americans remain committed to democracy.
    b. Americans are unwilling to fight in wars.
    c. America sustained losses in war.
    d. America needs to focus on itself.

This is true, that the wisdom of all these latter times, in princes' affairs, is rather fine deliveries, and shiftings of dangers and mischiefs, when they are near, than solid and grounded courses to keep them aloof. But this is but to try masteries with fortune. And let men beware, how they neglect and suffer matter of trouble to be prepared; for no man can forbid the spark, nor tell whence it may come. The difficulties in princes' business are many and great; but the greatest difficulty, is often in their own mind. For it is common with princes (saith Tacitus) to will contradictories, Sunt plerumque regum voluntates vehementes, et inter se contrariae. For it is the solecism of power, to think to command the end, and yet not to endure the mean.

Kings have to deal with their neighbors, their wives, their children, their prelates or clergy, their nobles, their second-nobles or gentlemen, their merchants, their commons, and their men of war; and from all these arise dangers, if care and circumspection be not used.

21. What is the main idea of the passage?
    a. Rulers have a lot to fear.
    b. Princes and kings are really lucky.
    c. The greatest dangers come from outside the kingdom.
    d. The ruler's own mind is his greatest danger.

22. Which statement is not a detail from the passage?
    a. Care and circumspection can help protect the king.
    b. Merchants often cheat the king.
    c. Preparation for difficulties is important.
    d. Tacitus wrote that it is important to endure the mean.

23. What is the meaning of circumspection in the last paragraph?
    a. Spying
    b. Consideration
    c. Deceit
    d. Kindness

24. What is the author's primary purpose in writing this passage?
    a. To educate kings
    b. To discuss the problems of rule
    c. To talk about royal marriage
    d. To analyze monarchy

25. Which is the best summary of this passage?
    a. Princes and kings have many challenges.
    b. Rulers should be kind and merciful.
    c. Avoid tolerating anyone near you.
    d. Kings can do whatever they like.

I did not, when a slave, understand the deep meaning of those rude and apparently incoherent songs. I was myself within the circle; so that I neither saw nor heard as those without might see and hear. They told a tale of woe which was then altogether beyond my feeble comprehension; they were tones loud, long, and deep; they breathed the prayer and complaint of souls boiling over with the bitterest anguish. Every tone was a testimony against slavery, and a prayer to God for deliverance from chains. The hearing of those wild notes always depressed my spirit, and filled me with ineffable sadness. I have frequently found myself in tears while hearing them. The mere recurrence to those songs, even now, afflicts me; and while I am writing these lines, an expression of feeling has already found its way down my cheek. To those songs I trace my first glimmering conception of the dehumanizing character of slavery. I can never get rid of that conception. Those songs still follow me, to deepen my hatred of slavery, and quicken my sympathies for my brethren in bonds. If any one wishes to be impressed with the soul-killing effects of slavery, let him go to Colonel Lloyd's plantation, and, on allowance-day, place himself in the deep pine woods, and there let him, in silence, analyze the sounds that shall pass through the chambers of his soul,—and if he is not thus impressed, it will only be because "there is no flesh in his obdurate heart."

26. What is the main idea of the passage?
    a. The music of the slaves expressed the sadness and devastation of slavery.
    b. Slavery was bad.
    c. The narrator had been a slave.
    d. The origins of Blues music are found in slavery.

27. Which statement is not a detail from the passage?
    a. The narrator was a slave in Virginia.
    b. Slaves sang while they worked.
    c. The songs could be compared to prayers.
    d. Colonel Lloyd owned the plantation.

28. What is the meaning of <u>obdurate</u> in the last line of the paragraph?
    a. Angry
    b. Sad
    c. Happy
    d. Stubborn

29. What is the author's primary purpose in writing this passage?
    a. Writing a fictional story about slavery
    b. Sharing his own story
    c. Explaining why slavery is bad
    d. Convincing others that slavery was bad

30. Which is the best summary of this passage?
    a. The songs of slaves expressed their deep sadness and grief.
    b. Slaves sang while working in the fields.
    c. Plantation owners were immoral and unkind.
    d. The narrator escaped slavery through the Underground Railroad.

We are told nothing as to sacrificial and religious rites, and all else is omitted which does not provide material for artistic treatment. The so-called Northern Mythology, therefore, may be regarded as a precious relic of the beginning of Northern poetry, rather than as a representation of the religious beliefs of the Scandinavians, and these literary fragments bear many signs of the transitional stage wherein the confusion of the old and new faiths is easily apparent.

But notwithstanding the limitations imposed by long neglect it is possible to reconstruct in part a plan of the ancient Norse beliefs, and the general reader will derive much profit from Carlyle's illuminating study in "Heroes and Hero-worship." "A bewildering, inextricable jungle of delusions, confusions, falsehoods and absurdities, covering the whole field of Life!" he calls them, with all good reason. But he goes on to show, with equal truth, that at the soul of this crude worship of distorted nature was a spiritual force seeking expression. What we probe without reverence they viewed with awe, and not understanding it, straightway deified it, as all children have been apt to do in all stages of the world's history. Truly they were hero-worshippers after Carlyle's own heart, and skepticism had no place in their simple philosophy.

31. What is the main idea of the passage?
    a. We have a lot of evidence about Norse religion.
    b. Norse literature provides information on Norse beliefs.
    c. Norse beliefs can be loosely reconstructed.
    d. The Norse practiced religious sacrifice.

32. Which statement is not a detail from the passage?
    a. Carlyle wrote about Norse beliefs.
    b. Scandinavian religion worshipped nature.
    c. Scandinavian literature reflects the transition from old to new religion.
    d. Nordic poetry is religious.

33. What is the meaning of skepticism near the end of the paragraph?
    a. Doubt
    b. Justification
    c. Faith
    d. Thought

34. What is the author's primary purpose in writing this passage?
    a. To introduce Norse religion
    b. To analyze Norse poetry
    c. To explain Norse history
    d. To introduce Norse culture

35. Which is the best summary of this passage?
    a. From what we know, the Norse religion was based around nature.
    b. The Norse worshipped heroes.
    c. Norse epics are about heroes.
    d. The Norse were successful conquerors.

Professor Murray will, I am sure, excuse me if I say that he has the common fault of most Englishmen of being inaudible. Why on earth people who have something to say which is worth hearing should not take the slight trouble to learn how to make it heard is one of the strange mysteries of modern life. Their methods are as reasonable as to try to pour some precious stuff from the spring to the reservoir through a non-conducting pipe, which could by the least effort be opened. Professor Murray made several profound remarks to his white tie and to the water-carafe upon the table, with a humorous, twinkling aside to the silver candlestick upon his right. Then he sat down, and Mr. Waldron, the famous popular lecturer, rose amid a general murmur of applause. He was a stern, gaunt man, with a harsh voice, and an aggressive manner, but he had the merit of knowing how to assimilate the ideas of other men, and to pass them on in a way which was intelligible and even interesting to the lay public, with a happy knack of being funny about the most unlikely objects, so that the precession of the Equinox or the formation of a vertebrate became a highly humorous process as treated by him.

36. What is the main idea of the passage?
     a. Public speaking is a useful skill.
     b. Mr. Waldron was a very good lecturer.
     c. Professor Murray talked to the water carafe.
     d. Lectures can be entertaining.

37. Which statement is not a detail from the passage?
     a. Mr. Waldron is a lecturer.
     b. Professor Murray cannot be heard.
     c. There is a silver candlestick.
     d. Mr. Waldron is quite jolly.

38. What is the meaning of <u>assimilate</u> near the end of the paragraph?
     a. Take in
     b. Dispute
     c. Agree with
     d. Overrule

39. What is the author's primary purpose in writing this passage?
     a. To educate
     b. To inform
     c. To entertain
     d. To argue

40. Which is the best summary of this passage?
     a. Mr. Waldron's lecture was more appealing than Professor Murray.
     b. Professor Murray could not be heard.
     c. Mr. Waldron was funny.
     d. Professor Murray looked down at the table.

"What are you doing there?" asked the Princess.
"I am spinning, my pretty child," answered the old woman, who did not know who she was.
"Oh, how pretty it is!" exclaimed the Princess. "How do you do it? Give it to me, that I may see if I can do it as well."

She had no sooner taken hold of the spindle, than, being very hasty, and rather thoughtless, and moreover, the fairies having ordained that it should be so, she pierced her hand with the point of it, and fainted away. The poor old woman was in great distress, and called for help. People came running from all quarters; they threw water in the Princess's face, they unlaced her dress, they slapped her hands, they rubbed her temples with Queen of Hungary's water, but nothing would bring her to. The King, who had run upstairs at the noise, then remembered the prediction of the fairies, and wisely concluded that this accident must have happened as the fairies had said it would. He ordered the Princess to be carried into a beautiful room of the palace, and laid on a bed embroidered with silver and gold. One might have thought it was an angel lying there, so lovely did she look, for the rich colors of her complexion had not faded in her swoon; her cheeks were still rosy, and her lips like coral. Only, her eyes were closed, but they could hear her breathing softly, which showed that she was not dead.

The King gave orders that she was to be left to sleep there in quiet, until the hour of her awaking should arrive. The good fairy who had saved her life, by condemning her to sleep for a hundred years, was in the Kingdom of Mataquin, twelve thousand leagues away, when the Princess met with her accident, but she was informed of it instantly by a little dwarf, who had a pair of seven-league boots, that is, boots which enabled the wearer to take seven leagues at a stride.

41. What is the main idea of the passage?
   a. The dwarf could take seven leagues at a stride.
   b. The fairies had condemned her to sleep.
   c. The princess pricked her finger and was cursed.
   d. The princess did not die.

42. Which statement is not a detail from the passage?
   a. A fairy saved the princess' life.
   b. The princess was cursed by Maleficient.
   c. The princess touched a spindle.
   d. A dwarf told the fairy what had happened.

43. What is the meaning of ordained in the second paragraph?
   a. Ordered
   b. Planned
   c. Allowed
   d. Disallowed

44. What is the author's primary purpose in writing this passage?
   a. To share a historical incident
   b. To entertain
   c. To educate
   d. To warn people about the danger of spindles

45. Which is the best summary of this passage?
   a. The princess was cursed and would sleep for 100 years.
   b. The prince needed to save the princess.
   c. Fairies are evil.
   d. The king was unkind and a poor ruler.

I could not perhaps appeal to an audience more capable of appreciating the truth of these remarks than to the members of an Institution, the object of which is to examine into the improvements and so-called inventions which are from time to time effected in the machinery and implements of war.

How often does any proposal or improvement come before this Institution which after investigating its antecedents is found to possess originality of design? Is it not a fact that even the most ingenious and successful inventions turn out on inquiry to be mere adaptations of contrivances already existing, or that they are produced by applying to one branch of industry the principles or the contrivances which have been evolved in another. I think that no one can have constantly attended the lectures of this or any similar Institution, without becoming impressed, above all things, with the want of originality observable amongst men, and with the great calls which, even in this age of cultivated intellects and abundant materials to work upon, all inventors are obliged to make upon those who have preceded them.

46. What is the main idea of the passage?
    a. There is little that is truly original.
    b. War has not changed.
    c. Implements of war require new materials.
    d. Ingenious inventions are entirely new.

47. Which statement is not a detail from the passage?
    a. The institution examines war implements.
    b. Inventions in one industry can be used in another.
    c. Inventors create entirely new items.
    d. Inventions build upon what came before.

48. What is the meaning of <u>antecedents</u> in the second paragraph?
    a. What came after
    b. What came before
    c. Other's ideas
    d. Plagiarism

49. What is the author's primary purpose in writing this passage?
    a. To introduce his topic
    b. To educate the audience
    c. To persuade the audience
    d. To show why his invention is better

50. Which is the best summary of this passage?
    a. Inventions and innovations build upon what came before them.
    b. New inventions are essential to industry.
    c. War supports innovation.
    d. Innovation stops during times of war.

Reading Section Practice Test #1 – ANSWER KEY

1.	B	26.	A
2.	D	27.	A
3.	A	28.	D
4.	D	29.	B
5.	A	30.	A
6.	B	31.	C
7.	D	32.	D
8.	D	33.	A
9.	A	34.	A
10.	B	35.	A
11.	C	36.	B
12.	A	37.	D
13.	B	38.	A
14.	A	39.	C
15.	D	40.	A
16.	C	41.	C
17.	A	42.	B
18.	B	43.	A
19.	C	44.	B
20.	A	45.	A
21.	D	46.	A
22.	B	47.	C
23.	B	48.	B
24.	B	49.	A
25.	A	50.	A

GRAMMAR SECTION PRACTICE TEST #1

1. Which word is a conjunction? We went to the grocery store, stopped for coffee, and picked up our dry cleaning.
   a. Our
   b. For
   c. And
   d. To

2. Select the best word or phrase for the blank. You need to get up now in order ___ make it to class on time.
   a. For
   b. To
   c. When
   d. Of

3. Which of the following is grammatically incorrect?
   a. Who goes to school on South Street.
   b. The boy goes to school on South Street.
   c. The girl attends the South Street School.
   d. Which of the children go to school on South Street?

4. Which is correct?
   a. The boy started school yesterday.
   b. The boy starts school yesterday.
   c. The boy started school tomorrow.
   d. The boy did start school tomorrow.

5. Select the best word or phrase for the blank. Please _____ your mom today.
   a. Calling
   b. Calls
   c. Called
   d. Call

6. Which word is a conjunction? Did you go to class or did you stay home sick today?
   a. Did
   b. Stay
   c. Today
   d. Or

7. Select the best word or phrase for the blank. The flight _____, so we will have to wait at the airport.
   a. Delays
   b. Delayed
   c. Is delayed
   d. Will delay

8. Which of the following is grammatically incorrect?
   a. Monitors track the patient's heart rate and oxygen levels.
   b. Monitor track the patient's heart rate and oxygen levels.
   c. You should carefully monitor the patients' vital signs.
   d. Watch the monitors from the nurses' station.

9. Which is correct?
   a. I need to do my homework now, so I can go to the movie now.
   b. I need to do my homework now, so I cannot go to the movie now.
   c. I need to doing my homework now, so I cannot go to the movie now.
   d. I need to do my homework now, so I cannot going to the movie now.

10. Which word is a noun? The puppy's favorite toy is pink and fuzzy.
    a. Pink
    b. Fuzzy
    c. Favorite
    d. Toy

11. Which word is a noun? The bell will ring in five minutes.
    a. Minutes
    b. Five
    c. Will
    d. Ring

12. Which is correct?
    a. You can have either the cake nor the cookie.
    b. You can't have neither the cake or the cookie.
    c. You can have either the cake or the cookie.
    d. You can having either the cake or the cookie.

13. Which word or phrase is a preposition? Put the groceries on the table, please.
    a. Table
    b. Put
    c. Please
    d. On

14. Which word or phrase is a preposition? He checked into the hospital early that morning for his surgery.
    a. Checked
    b. He
    c. Into
    d. Hospital

15. Which is correct?
    a. Who is going to class on Saturday.
    b. Who is goes to class on Saturday?
    c. Whose going to class on Saturday?
    d. Who is going to class on Saturday?

16. Which word or phrase is the subject? After the children finished painting, they had to clean up their mess.
    a. Mess
    b. Painting
    c. Finished
    d. They

17. Which word or phrase is the subject? She popped popcorn, grabbed a drink and sat down to watch her favorite show.
    a. She
    b. Popcorn
    c. Drink
    d. Show

18. Select the best word or phrase for the blank. _____ you want to work in home health care after graduation?
    a. Does
    b. Do
    c. Was
    d. Did

19. Which of the following is grammatically incorrect?
    a. I work on the maternity floor at the hospital.
    b. I work in maternity at the hospital.
    c. I works on the maternity floor at the hospital.
    d. I work in maternity at the hospital.

20. Select the best word or phrase for the blank. She _____ a doctor's appointment in the morning, so she was late to work that day.
    a. Has
    b. Had
    c. Will have
    d. Was

21. Which is correct?
    a. The baby is due in December.
    b. The baby dues in December.
    c. The babies is due in December.
    d. The baby are due in December.

22. Which word is the direct object? She finished decorating the kitchen for the party early that morning.
    a. Morning
    b. She
    c. Kitchen
    d. Early

23. Which word is the direct object? He was scheduled to work a 12-hour shift.
    a. Shift
    b. He
    c. 12-hour
    d. Work

24. Which is correct?
    a. I learned to write good working at the paper.
    b. I learned to write well working at the paper.
    c. I teached to write well working at the paper.
    d. I learned to write well working to the paper.

25. Which of the following is grammatically incorrect?
    a. The librarian at the reference desk is very helpful.
    b. The reference desk librarian is very helpful.
    c. Is the reference desk librarian helpful?
    d. Can the reference desk librarian helpful?

26. Which is the dependent clause? Do you know the librarian who works on Saturday mornings?
    a. Do you know
    b. The librarian
    c. Saturday mornings
    d. Who works on Saturday mornings

27. Which is the dependent clause? I like to cook, which is good since I work in a restaurant.
    a. Like to cook
    b. I like to
    c. Which is good since I work in a restaurant
    d. I work in a restaurant

28. Which is correct?
    a. The baseball game was cancelled because of rain.
    b. The baseball game will cancelled because of rain.
    c. The baseball game was cancel because of rain.
    d. The baseball games was cancelled because to rain.

29. Which word or phrase is the predicate? The boy threw the ball across the field.
    a. The boy
    b. Threw the ball across the field
    c. Across the field
    d. The boy threw the ball

30. Which of the following is grammatically incorrect?
    a. The dance was scheduled for next Saturday night.
    b. The dance is scheduled for next Saturday night.
    c. Schedule the dance for next Saturday night.
    d. Scheduling the dance for next Saturday night.

31. Which word or phrase is the predicate? Michelle and her dog walk in the park every day.
    a. Michelle
    b. Michelle and her dog
    c. Walk in the park every day
    d. In the park every day

32. Which is correct?
    a. I heard about the plane crash on the news.
    b. I read about the plane crash on the news.
    c. I heard on the plane crash on the news.
    d. I hear about the plane crash to the news.

33. Which has a predicate adjective?
    a. Dinner smells amazing.
    b. We are going to dinner.
    c. He ate a sandwich.
    d. The car has a leak in the radiator.

34. Which has a predicate adjective?
    a. The doctor is concerned about her symptoms.
    b. I scheduled an appointment.
    c. I have to work on Tuesday.
    d. He bought a new phone.

35. Choose the best substitute for the underlined word. I have a class on Mondays at 4:00 PM and have to prepare the lecture before class and speak with students after class.
    a. Take
    b. Learn
    c. Teach
    d. Attend

36. Which of the following is grammatically incorrect?
    a. Nurses may work in the home, doctor's office or hospital.
    b. Nurses works in the home, doctor's office or hospital.
    c. Nurses can work in the home, doctor's office or hospital.
    d. Nurses may work in either the home, doctor's office or hospital.

37. Choose the best substitute for the underlined word. The ambulance took the patient to the hospital after he called 911.
    a. Brought
    b. Transferred
    c. Carried
    d. Went

38. Select the word used incorrectly. He swimmed across the lake last summer.
    a. Across
    b. Lake
    c. Swimmed
    d. Summer

39. Select the word used incorrectly. Neither the dog or the cat like going to the vet.
    a. Neither
    b. Like
    c. Going
    d. Or

40. Select the best word or phrase for the blank. I _____ never going to work there.
    a. Am not
    b. Will
    c. Will not
    d. Am

41. Which of the following is grammatically incorrect?
    a. Take the patient into the examining room.
    b. Takes the patient into the examining room.
    c. You should take the patient into the examining room.
    d. He takes the patient into the examining room.

42. The following contains which type of phrase? The butcher, who has his own shop, is known for the quality of his meat.
    a. Prepositional phrase
    b. Predicate adjective
    c. Dependent clause
    d. Conjunction

43. Select the best word or phrase for the blank. _____ you planning to attend the meeting?
    a. Is
    b. Are
    c. Will
    d. Was

44. Which of the following is grammatically incorrect?
    a. I checked the patient's vital signs and entered them into the computer.
    b. I changed into scrubs at the beginning of my shift.
    c. The patient, who had surgery that day, was nervous.
    d. The patients was prepped for surgery that morning.

45. The following contains which type of phrase? We are baking cookies to take to the school bake sale.
    a. Dependent clause
    b. Prepositional phrase
    c. Predicate adjective
    d. Contraction

46. Select the best word or phrase for the blank. Can you _____ on the patient in room 302?
    a. Watch
    b. Check
    c. Talk
    d. Care

47. Select the best word or phrase for the blank. She was scared ___ spiders, so avoided the basement.
    a. To
    b. For
    c. Of
    d. From

48. Select the best word or phrase for the blank. They were _____ for a new car to purchase.
    a. Looks
    b. Looking
    c. Wanting
    d. Shops

49. Select the best word or phrase for the blank. I am waiting _____ the bus.
    a. For
    b. To
    c. Catch
    d. Catching

50. Select the best word or phrase for the blank. I _____ overtime this week, so cannot go out tonight.
    a. Will work
    b. Work
    c. Working
    d. Works

Grammar Practice Test #1 – ANSWER KEY

1. C And is a conjunction, joining two things.

2. B To is the correct choice.

3. A Option A is a question, but has no question mark.

4. A Yesterday implies past tense, so started is the correct verb choice.

5. D The implied subject is you, tense is present, so call is correct.

6. D Or, joining two parts of the sentence, is a conjunction.

7. C Present passive is the best choice here, so is delayed.

8. B Subject and verb do not match and there is a missing apostrophe in patient's

9. B If you have to do your homework, you cannot attend a movie at the same time.

10. D Toy, as a noun is a person, place or thing.

11. A Minutes, a noun is a person, place or thing.

12. C Either has to go with or. Option D has a verb error.

13. D On is a preposition.

14. C Into is a preposition.

15. D Option A does not have a question mark, B has a verb error and C uses the possessive whose.

16. D The first part of the sentence is a clause, they, referring to the children, is the subject.

17. A She is the one who did everything or the subject.

18. B Do is correct. Does requires a third person subject, was a first person and did is past tense.

19. C Subject and verb do not match.

20. B The appointment has already happened, so had, or the past tense is correct.

21. A Subject and verb agree.

22. C Kitchen is the direct object, or the thing being decorated.

23. A Shift is the direct object.

24. B I learned to write well working at the paper is the only correct option. A has an incorrect adjective, C an incorrect verb and D an incorrect preposition.

25. D D is incorrect as can requires a verb, not an adjective, like helpful.

26. D Who works on Saturday mornings is the dependent clause. It cannot stand alone as a statement.

27. C Which is good… is a dependent clause, unable to stand on its own in a statement.

28. A B & C have verb errors, while D has a preposition error.

29. B The predicate is the verb plus anything following.

30. D D is a sentence fragment, lacking a subject

31. C The predicate is the verb plus anything following.

32. A C and D use incorrect prepositions. B is technically correct; however, on the news implies heard, rather than read.

33. A A predicate adjective directly describes the subject of the sentence.

34. A A predicate adjective directly describes the subject of the sentence.

35. C The context of the sentence makes it clear that the speaker is the teacher of the class.

36. B The subject and verb do not agree.

37. A Brought is the best substitute.

38. C Swam is the past tense of swim.

39. D Neither goes with nor not or.

40. D Am is correct. Will does not agree with the verb tense and the others produce a double negative.

41. B The verb does not agree with the implied subject, you.

42. C Who has his own shop is a dependent clause.

43. B Are is the only one that agrees with the subject and the planning to attend.

44. D Subject and verb disagree.

45. B To take to the school bake sale is a prepositional phrase.

46. B Only "check" can be paired with the word "on".

47. C Of is the only correct response when paired with "scared".

48. B Looking is the only choice that works with both were and for.

49. A For is correct. Catch would require the addition of to.

50. B Work is correct, present tense construction.

VOCABULARY PRACTICE TEST #1

1. Which of the following statements uses a euphemism?
    a. He passed away last week.
    b. He died yesterday.
    c. The baby was born last month.
    d. The dog ran away, but was found after two days.

2. Saving money may be smart, but she thought he was too frugal. Select the meaning of the underlined word.
    a. Wealthy
    b. Poor
    c. Thrifty
    d. Lavish

3. Which word means happiness?
    a. Exemplary
    b. Exuberance
    c. Excitement
    d. Expansion

4. Their divorce was especially acrimonious. Select the meaning of the underlined word.
    a. Easy
    b. Lengthy
    c. Pleasant
    d. Bitter

5. Which of the following words is a synonym of sad?
    a. Morose
    b. Acerbic
    c. Irate
    d. Jovial

6. Which of these words is not spelled correctly?
    a. Affect
    b. Loose
    c. Definately
    d. Irritable

7. What is the best description of they're?
    a. Contraction
    b. Conjunction
    c. Preposition
    d. Subject

8. What is the best description of <u>quickly</u>?
   a. Adjective
   b. Interjection
   c. Adverb
   d. Verb

9. Which word that means hurried best fits? She didn't want to be late, so she _____ to work.
   a. Scurried
   b. Accelerated
   c. Expedited
   d. Rushed

10. Select the word or phrase that will be grammatically correct. They completed _____ homework on time.
    a. There
    b. They're
    c. Their
    d. Them

11. What is the best description of <u>upon</u>?
    a. Noun
    b. Preposition
    c. Adjective
    d. Subjective

12. Which word means <u>slow</u>?
    a. Languid
    b. Agitated
    c. Hastened
    d. Unmoving

13. Select the correct order of words.
    a. The old car was in the shop for repairs.
    b. For repairs, the old car was in the shop.
    c. The car old was for repairs in the shop.
    d. In the shop, the old car was for repairs.

14. The lecture was <u>ponderous</u> and many of the students found themselves dozing off during class. Select the meaning of the underlined word.
    a. Interesting
    b. Boring
    c. Exciting
    d. Difficult

15. Which word that means <u>young</u> fits best in this sentence? The _____ animals learned to hunt alongside their mothers.
    a. Immature
    b. Naïve
    c. Baby
    d. Juvenile

16. Which word is not spelled correctly?
    a. Alot
    b. Allot
    c. Allocate
    d. Allotment

17. Select the meaning of the underlined word. The holiday bonuses were a <u>boon</u> for many families.
    a. Loss
    b. Challenge
    c. Joy
    d. Blessing

18. Which word that means angry best fits the sentence? He was _____ after being cut off in traffic.
    a. Irate
    b. Annoyed
    c. Indignant
    d. Apoplectic

19. Select the word or phrase that will be grammatically correct. _____ best friend's birthday is tomorrow.
    a. Your
    b. You are
    c. You're
    d. The

20. Which word means <u>learned</u>?
    a. Absorbed
    b. Taught
    c. Remembered
    d. Acquainted

21. Which word is not spelled correctly?
    a. Argument
    b. Arguement
    c. Agreement
    d. Aggravation

22. Which word is not spelled correctly?
    a. Judgment
    b. Judgement
    c. Judiciary
    d. Judicial

23. Which word is not a synonym for excited?
    a. Exhilarated
    b. Enthusiastic
    c. Thrilled
    d. Exhausted

24. Select the meaning of the underlined word. He was anxious about the test results.
    a. Angry
    b. Sad
    c. Happy
    d. Worried

25. Select the word or phrase that will be grammatically correct in the sentence. The child was _____ cold, so he asked his mother for his jacket.
    a. Very
    b. Not
    c. Too much
    d. Not much

26. Select the correct order of words.
    a. She wanted him to read her a story.
    b. She wanted to read a story by him.
    c. She wanted her a story read by him.
    d. She wanted a read story by him.

27. Which word is not spelled correctly?
    a. Pharmacy
    b. Medical
    c. Medecine
    d. Medication

28. Which word means mistake?
    a. Error
    b. Correction
    c. Accuracy
    d. Review

29. Select the word or phrase that will be grammatically correct? I've been in nursing school _____ six months.
    a. Since
    b. After
    c. Before
    d. For

30. Which word is a synonym for <u>tired</u>?
    a. Energetic
    b. Driven
    c. Fatigued
    d. Melancholy

31. Select the correct order of words:
    a. Into the hospital, checked the patient.
    b. The patient checked into the hospital.
    c. Checked into the hospital the patient.
    d. The hospital checked into the patient.

32. Which word means illness?
    a. Injury
    b. Ailment
    c. Irritation
    d. Symptom

33. Which word is a synonym for <u>disease</u>?
    a. Infection
    b. Malady
    c. Seizure
    d. Hemorrhage

34. Select the word or phrase that will be grammatically correct. The doctor _____ the patient yesterday on rounds.
    a. Seen
    b. Saw
    c. Sees
    d. Will see

35. Select the meaning of the underlined word. <u>Tardiness </u>is not tolerated, and you will be counted absent.
    a. Illness
    b. Absence
    c. Lateness
    d. Attendance

36. Which of the following words is a synonym of <u>contagious</u>?
    a. Transmissible
    b. Poisonous
    c. Non-communicable
    d. Venereal

37. Select the meaning of the underlined word. The staff was concerned about a <u>rash</u> of flu cases at the hospital.
    a. Epidemic
    b. Irritation
    c. Disease
    d. Symptom

38. Select the meaning of the underlined word. The patient complained of <u>bilateral</u> weakness.
    a. Right side
    b. Left side
    c. Both sides
    d. Upper body

39. Select the meaning of the underlined word. Since the two could not get along at the office, they were referred for <u>mediation</u>.
    a. Relaxation
    b. Medication
    c. Arbitration
    d. Arguments

40. Select the meaning of the underlined word. Careful hand washing is an essential <u>precaution</u> in the workplace.
    a. Preventative
    b. Cause
    c. Carelessness
    d. Rule

41. Select the meaning of the underlined word. The change in the patient's condition was <u>sudden</u>.
    a. Slow
    b. Unnoticeable
    c. Unexpected
    d. Significant

42. Select the meaning of the underlined word. Many medical tests should be scheduled <u>annually</u>.
    a. Every year
    b. Every month
    c. Every other year
    d. Every decade

43. Select the meaning of the underlined word. Chest congestion may be <u>audible</u> when you examine the patient.
    a. Severe
    b. Able to be heard
    c. Mild
    d. Able to be seen

44. Select the meaning of the underlined word. In many cases, the other senses can <u>compensate</u> for the loss of one sense.
    a. Worsen
    b. Improve
    c. Offset
    d. Acclimate

45. Select the meaning of the underlined word. Bronchitis and ear infections are possible <u>complications</u> of the common cold.
    a. Developments
    b. Benefits
    c. Infections
    d. Panaceas

46. Select the meaning of the underlined word. When you're cooking, it's important to get the <u>consistency</u> of the sauce correct.
    a. Color
    b. Shape
    c. Viscosity
    d. Fluidity

47. Select the meaning of the underlined word. Allergies are a possible <u>contraindication</u> for some medications.
    a. Prescription
    b. Reason
    c. Reason not to take
    d. Medical need

48. Select the meaning of the underlined word. Vitamin and mineral <u>deficiencies</u> can cause a number of symptoms.
    a. Insufficiencies
    b. Abundance
    c. Excess
    d. Tablets

49. Select the meaning of the underlined word. The patient complains that his symptoms are <u>worsening</u>.
    a. Improving
    b. Gone
    c. Deteriorating
    d. Changing

50. Select the meaning of the underlined word. The pupils should <u>dilate</u> in low light.
    a. Expand
    b. Decrease
    c. Brighten
    d. Shine

Vocabulary Practice Test #1 – ANSWER KEY

1. A Euphemisms are a more polite way to say something, like passed away in place of died.
2. C
3. B
4. D
5. A
6. C The correct spelling is definitely.
7. A They're is a contraction of they are.
8. C Quickly, like other words ending in –ly, is an adverb.
9. D
10. C Their is the correct, possessive form.
11. B Upon is a preposition.
12. A
13. A The old car was in the shop for repairs. The adjective, old, comes before the noun it modifies, while in the shop describes where the car was.
14. B
15. D
16. A Alot should be a lot.
17. D
18. B
19. A
20. A
21. B Arguement should be argument.
22. B Judgement should be judgment.
23. D
24. D
25. A
26. A She wanted him to read her a story is correct. She is the subject, wanted the verb, and him the direct object.
27. C Medecine should be medicine.
28. A
29. D She has been in nursing school for six months. Has been implies both past tense and continuance.
30. C
31. B The patient is the subject, checked the verb, and into the hospital a prepositional phrase.
32. B
33. B
34. B The doctor saw the patient yesterday on rounds. Yesterday shows that this   will be past tense.
35. C
36. A
37. A
38. C
39. C
40. A
41. C
42. A

43. B
44. C
45. A
46. C
47. C
48. A
49. C
50. A

BIOLOGY PRACTICE TEST #1

1. Which of the following is true regarding deoxyribonucleic acid (DNA) in the human body?
   A. DNA is used as an energy source.
   B. DNA is used as a template for creation of proteins.
   C. DNA is only found in the brain.
   D. DNA is made of sugar.

2. Testes are an organ found in:
   A. Females
   B. Plants
   C. Males
   D. Amoebas

3. How many kingdoms of life are there?
   A. 3
   B. 6
   C. 7
   D. 9

4. Plants absorb carbon dioxide (CO_2) to create sugar for energy. What is the primary byproduct of this process?
   A. Oxygen
   B. Nitrogen
   C. Carbon Monoxide
   D. Carbon

5. What prevents ultraviolet radiation produced by the sun from damaging life on earth?
   A. The ozone layer
   B. Greenhouse gases
   C. The vacuum between earth and the sun
   D. The water layer

6. Which of the following is *not* present in an animal cell?
   A. Nucleus
   B. Mitochondria
   C. Cytoplasm
   D. Cell Wall

7. Mitosis is the process of cell division to create new cells. What is the process of cell division required to create new sex cells, or gametes?

   A. Telosis
   B. Meiosis
   C. Kinesis
   D. Phoresis

8. What are the two main parts of the human body's central nervous system?

   A. The heart and the spinal cord
   B. The brain and the spinal cord
   C. The peripheral nerves and the brain
   D. The spinal cord and the peripheral nerves

9. Which of the following is not an organ system in humans?

   A. The endocrine system
   B. The respiratory system
   C. The exophatic system
   D. The muscular system

10. Humans can turn glucose into ATP, the basic energy molecule in the body. What is a byproduct of this process?

    A. Carbon dioxide
    B. Oxygen
    C. Nitrogen
    D. Phosphorus

11. Which of the following is not in the Kingdom Plantae?

    A. Cactus
    B. Algae
    C. Oak Tree
    D. Sunflower

12. What is the primary difference between a cell membrane and a cell wall?

    A. A cell membrane is flexible and a cell wall is rigid.
    B. A cell membrane is not found in plants, whereas a cell wall is.
    C. A cell membrane is not found in animals, whereas a cell wall is.
    D. A cell membrane is composed of protein, whereas a cell wall is composed of sugar.

13. Plants are autotrophs, meaning that they:

    A. Consume organic material produced by animals
    B. They produce their own food
    C. They are able to move by themselves
    D. They can automatically transform from a seed into a plant.

14. Which of the following is *not* true of a virus?
    A. Viruses have DNA
    B. Viruses do not have a nucleus
    C. Viruses cannot survive without water
    D. Viruses can be infectious

15. In the digestive system, the majority of nutrients are absorbed in the:
    A. Esophagus
    B. Stomach
    C. Small Intestine
    D. Large Intestine

16. Which of the following kingdom's members have tissue called hyphae?

    a) Fungi.
    b) Animalia.
    c) Protista.
    d) Plantae.

17. Which organelle is important in the production of polysaccharides (carbohydrates)?

    e) Mitochondrion.
    f) Golgi apparatus.
    g) Nucleus
    h) Endoplasmic reticulum.

18. In humans, DNA is compressed into larger bodies called:
    A. Chromosomes
    B. Histones
    C. Barr Bodies
    D. None of the above

19. Which of the following statements is *not* true regarding RNA?
    A. RNA is produced from a transcript of DNA
    B. RNA is read by a ribosome to produce proteins
    C. RNA is non-degradable and exists permanently in the cell
    D. RNA uses uracil rather than thymine as a nucleotide

20. In DNA replication, what enzyme is responsible for copying the DNA?
    A. DNA helicase
    B. DNA polymerase
    C. DNA transcriptase
    D. DNA replicase

21. After two haploid cells a result of meiosis combine, they become a:
    A. Diploid zygote
    B. Haploid gamete
    C. Diploid morula
    D. Haploid blastosphere

22. In meiosis,
    A. The amount of DNA stays the same in all stages
    B. The end product has genes evenly split between mother and father
    C. The process results in 4 cells instead of two
    D. The period of metaphase is shorter than in that of mitosis

23. The RNA strand AUGCACAGG codes for which sequence of amino acids?
    A. M-H-V
    B. V-H-R
    C. M-H-R
    D. R-A-V

24. An exon coding for a protein was found to be 63 base pairs in length. This protein would contain:
    A. 12 amino acids
    B. 21 amino acids
    C. 27 amino acids
    D. 60 amino acids

25. Which of the following is a difference between eukaryotic and prokaryotic DNA transcription?
    A. DNA transcription only occurs in eukaryotic cells.
    B. In prokaryotic cells, the mRNA is read by a complex called a spliceosome, not a ribosome.
    C. In eukaryotic cells, DNA is transcribed by DNA polymerase, not RNA polymerase.
    D. None of the above is a difference.

Biology Practice Test #1 Answer Key

1. B
2. C
3. B
4. A
5. A
6. D
7. B
8. B
9. C
10. A
11. B
12. A
13. B
14. C
15. C
16. A
17. B
18. A
19. C
20. B
21. A
22. C
23. C
24. B
25. D

CHEMISTRY PRACTICE TEST #1

1. A student calculates that there are 1.5 mols of gas in a sample volume he has collected. How many molecules of gas are there?
    a) 6.022×10^{23}
    b) 9.033×10^{-23}
    c) 9.033×10^{23}
    d) 6.02214×10^{24}

2. The average adult human male weighs about 70 kg. How many grams is this?
    a) 70×10^5 grams
    b) 7.0×10^2 grams
    c) 7.0×10^5 grams
    d) 3.5×10^4 grams

3. The national debt of the United States at the start of 2014 is $17,419,636,128,544.61. Convert this to scientific notation.
    a) 17.419×10^8
    b) 17.42×10^{12}
    c) 1.741×10^{13}
    d) 1.743×10^{12}

4. What is the metric unit to measure mass?
    a) Kilojoule
    b) Calorie
    c) Pound
    d) Gram

5. A student finds out that gravity on the moon is ½ that of Earth. If he weighs 60 kg on Earth, how much will he weigh on the moon?
    a) 66.13 lbs
    b) 66.13 kg
    c) 35 kg
    d) 120.5 lbs

6. The average temperatures in June, July and August were 27 °C, 29 °C and 31 °C, respectively. What was the average temperature across the three months?
    a) 27 °C
    b) 28 °C
    c) 29 °C
    d) 30 °C

7. A refrigerator commonly stores goods at 4 °C, or:
    a) 39 °F
    b) 42 °F
    c) 299 K
    d) 350 K

8. The sun is estimated to have a surface temperature of around 5778 K, which is pretty darn hot. Would this be enough to melt tungsten, which has a melting point of 6191 °F?
   a) Yes, but not by much.
   b) Yes, more than hot enough.
   c) No, needs to be a little hotter.
   d) No, the sun's temperature isn't even close.

9. A teaspoon of dry coffee crystals dissolves when mixed in a cup of hot water. This process produces a coffee solution. The original crystals are classified as a:
   c) Solute.
   d) Solvent.
   e) Reactant.
   f) Product.

10. Which of the following is likely to have the most number of molecules?
    a) 1 liter of water vapor
    b) 1 liter of water
    c) 0.5 liters of ice
    d) 0.5 liters of an ice water mixture

11. Which of the following is *not* true about a liquid?
    a) A liquid can always be compressed.
    b) A liquid is fluid and can change shape.
    c) A liquid is higher in energy than a solid.
    d) Molecules in a liquid can have attractive interactions.

12. Which of these is not a solid?
    a) Hair
    b) A fork
    c) Orange juice
    d) A desk

13. The freezing point of a compound is:
    a) The same as the boiling point of the compound
    b) The same as melting point of the compound
    c) The same as the triple point of the compound
    d) The same as the critical point of the compound

14. Which of these is the only state of matter in which molecules are not typically moving?
    a) Gas
    b) Liquid
    c) Plasma
    d) Solid

15. When a liquid turns into a gas, it is known as vaporization. What is the opposite process?
   a) Condensation
   b) Sublimation
   c) Transmogrification
   d) Precipitation

16. Liquids that are highly viscous, such as grease or paint, are:
   a) Resistant to movement
   b) Highly flammable
   c) Able to become solid at high temperatures
   d) None of the above

17. Fluorine, chlorine, and bromine are all very reactive. This is because they have:
   a) 2 S-shell electrons
   b) 7 valence electrons
   c) A very large electron shell
   d) None of the above

18. If magnesium has 13 neutrons, how many protons does it have?
   a) 12
   b) 13
   c) 14
   d) 11

19. A scientist has isolated Fe (III), a variant of iron that has a charge of 3+. Which of the following compounds could be created from this element?
   a) FeO_2
   b) $FeCl$
   c) $FeCa_3$
   d) Fe_2O_3

20. What is the VSEPR structure of a PO_4 (phosphate) molecule?
   a) Tetrahedral
   b) Octahedral
   c) Linear
   d) Trigonal biplanar

21. A double bond between two atoms, for example the double bond between oxygen in O_2, has how many electrons?
   a) 2
   b) 4
   c) 6
   d) 8

22. The specific heat of ethanol is about 2.3 J/g*K. If you want to heat 100g of ethanol from 25 °C until its boiling point, and have it all be vaporized, how much energy do you need?
    a) 545 kJ
    b) 977 kJ
    c) 129 kJ
    d) 822 kJ

23. A 50 liter volume of water vapor is condensed into liquid. Approximately how much volume will the liquid be?
    a) Less than 50 mL
    b) Between 50 mL and 200 mL
    c) About 1 liter
    d) More than 1 liter

24. When you notice that a chemical reaction equation is not balanced stoichiometrically, which of the following can be performed to balance the equation?
    a) Change the formula of the products
    b) Change the subscripts of the molecular formulas
    c) Change the coefficients of the reactants or products
    d) Change the reaction type

25. A scientist places mercury oxide (HgO) into a sealed chamber and heats it to 400 °C, causing a reaction to occur. When she opens the chamber, she notices liquid mercury has formed as well as oxygen gas. This reaction is a:
    a) Endothermic synthesis reaction
    b) Exothermic combustion reaction
    c) Endothermic decomposition reaction
    d) Exothermic replacement reaction

CHEMISTRY PRACTICE TEST #1 – ANSWER KEY

1. C
2. C
3. C
4. D
5. A
6. C
7. A
8. B
9. A
10. B
11. A
12. C
13. B
14. D
15. A
16. A
17. B
18. A
19. D
20. A
21. B
22. C
23. A
24. C
25. C

ANATOMY & PHYSIOLOGY PRACTICE TEST #1

1. Each alveolus in the lungs is covered by tiny blood vessels to perform which of these functions?
    a) Excretion of fluids.
    b) Gas exchange.
    c) Blood production.
    d) Air intake.

2. Which of the following occurs during gas exchange in a cell?
    a) Oxygen is flowing from a low concentration inside the cell to a high concentration outside the cell.
    b) Oxygen is flowing from a high concentration in the red blood cells to a low concentration inside the body cell.
    c) Carbon dioxide is moving from the red blood cells into the body cells, while oxygen is moving from the body cells into the red blood cells.
    d) Carbon dioxide is flowing from a low concentration outside the cells to a high concentration inside the cells.

3. Which of the following is NOT a function of the skeletal system in animals?
    a) Transport fluids.
    b) Produce oil.
    c) Placement of internal organs.
    d) Production of blood cells.

4. Which of the following is true of bones?
    a) They contain nerves.
    b) Some are unbreakable.
    c) They are present in vertebrates.
    d) They directly touch each other at a joint.

5. Which of the following animals does **NOT** have an exoskeleton?
    a) Insects.
    b) Crabs.
    c) Lobsters.
    d) Earthworms.

6. What type of tissue is found at joints and protects bones from rubbing against each other and becoming damaged?
    a) Contractile.
    b) Connective.
    c) Conductive.
    d) Catabolic.

7. Chyme is:
    a) Water and completely broken down food molecules.
    b) Acids and completely broken down food molecules.
    c) Acids and partially broken down some food molecules.
    d) Water and partially broken down some food molecules.

8. Where is bile stored?
    a) In the pancreas.
    b) In the gallbladder.
    c) In the liver.
    d) In the small intestines.

9. Which of the following is NOT an accessory organ of the digestive system?
    a) Liver.
    b) Pancreas.
    c) Gall bladder.
    d) Urinary bladder.

10. What are the three types of muscle cells?
    a) Cardiac, synaptic, and skeletal.
    b) Cardiac, autonomic, and smooth.
    c) Skeletal, cardiac, and smooth.
    d) Smooth, cardiac, and spinal.

11. Which of the following is true about skeletal muscles?
    a) They all contract unconsciously.
    b) All muscle movement is consciously controlled.
    c) They connect directly to one another.
    d) They are also known as striated muscles.

12. Flagellum and cilia:
    a) Work with an organism's muscles for movement.
    b) Are parts of all cells and are required for movement.
    c) Are used by organisms without muscular systems.
    d) None of the above.

13. Which of the following is NOT one of the chambers in the four-chambered vertebrate heart?
    a) Right atrium.
    b) Right ventricle.
    c) Left alveolar.
    d) Left ventricle.

14. Which of the following is true about blood flow in the four-chambered vertebrate heart circulatory system?
    a) Blood in the pulmonary vein is oxygenated.
    b) Blood in the pulmonary artery is oxygenated.
    c) Blood in the aorta is not oxygenated.
    d) Blood in the vena cava is oxygenated.

15. Which of the following are the major components of blood?
- a) Proteins and lipids.
- b) Plasma and cells.
- c) Proteins and platelets.
- d) Dells and lipids.

16. Platelets perform which of the following functions?
- a) Blood clotting.
- b) Carrying oxygen.
- c) Carrying carbon dioxide.
- d) Disease protection.

17. Red blood cells perform which of the following functions?
- a) Blood clotting.
- b) Carrying oxygen and carbon dioxide.
- c) Disease protection.
- d) Wound healing.

18. The kidneys filter which of the following from blood?
- a) Undigested food.
- b) Metabolic wastes.
- c) Blood cells.
- d) Platelets.

19. The nephron is where _____ is produced.
- a) Urine.
- b) Ammonia.
- c) Nucleic acid.
- d) Amino acid.

20. Waste concentrated in the Bowman's capsule is called:
- a) Urine.
- b) Salts.
- c) Nucleic acids.
- d) Amino acids.

21. Alcohol consumption increases urination because it:
- a) Increases the amount of water in the body.
- b) Increases the action of antidiuretic hormone.
- c) Decreases the action of antidiuretic hormone.
- d) Stops water reabsorption.

22. What is the chemical substance that carries a message from one cell to another?
- a) Axon fluid.
- b) Dendrite fluid.
- c) Neurotransmitter.
- d) Hormone.

23. Dendrites receive information from:

    a) The axon of other neurons.

    b) The dendrites of other neurons.

    c) The cell body of other neurons.

    d) The nucleus of other neurons.

24. _____ release neurotransmitters.

    a) Axons.

    b) Dendrites.

    c) Cell bodies.

    d) The nucleus.

25. 10. What happens during ovulation?

    a) A mature egg is produced

    b) The endometrium shreds

    c) The zygote plants itself into the vulva

    d) None of the above

1. b)
2. b)
3. b)
4. c)
5. d)
6. b)
7. c)
8. b)
9. d)
10. c)
11. d)
12. c)
13. c)
14. a)
15. b)
16. a)
17. b)
18. b)
19. a)
20. a)
21. c)
22. c)
23. a)
24. a)
25. a)

PHYSICS PRACTICE TEST #1

1. Calculate the amount of work done in moving a mass of 10kg at rest with a force of 5N in 8 seconds with no repulsive forces in action?
   a) 80J
   b) 100J
   c) 120J
   d) 60J

2. Consider 3 equal masses at arbitrary points A, B & C in the space and let D be a point on the surface of the earth (as shown in figure).

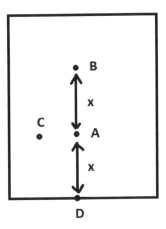

   Then,
   i. The mass at point B has the maximum potential energy
   ii. Masses at points A & C have equal P.E. but less than that of the mass at point D
   iii. The mass atpoint D, if lifted to a height 2x, will possess P.E. equal to P.E(B)
   a) Statements (i), (ii) & (iii) are true
   b) Only statements (i) & (iii) are true
   c) None of them is true
   d) Only statements (i) is true

3. The disc in the figure is set to rolled with angular velocity omega.

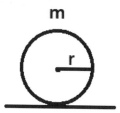

m

r

Total energy of the ball is:
a) $\frac{1}{2}mr^2w^2$
b) $\frac{3}{4}mrw^2$
c) $\frac{1}{2}mrw^2$
d) $\frac{3}{4}mr^2w^2$

4. Consider the following table:

S.No.	Length (cm)	Breadth (cm)
Wedge 1	5	2
Wedge 2	7	3
Wedge 3	4	6
Wedge 4	9	4

Which of the above wedges will provide maximum Mechanical Advantage?
a) Wedge 1
b) Wedge 2
c) Wedge 3
d) Wedge 4

5. A block P of mass 100kg is tied to one end of a rope on a frictionless pulley to lift another block Q with mass 40kg. What is the amount of acceleration produced in the rope during the lifting action?

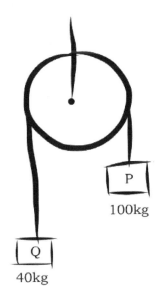

100kg

40kg

a) 2.4m/s²
b) 3.3m/s²
c) 4.2m/s²
d) 5.1m/s²

6. In the above problem, the value of acceleration [BH8]for block P & Q are:
a) Negative & Positive respectively
b) Positive & Negative respectively
c) Both Negative
d) Both Positive

7. A train of mass 100 tonnes is travelling with a uniform velocity of 108kmph. The driver is informed about a broken bridge 250m away from his present location. He immediately applies the brakes. If the coefficient of friction between the train and the rails is 0.2, what is the uniform deceleration[BH9] achieved by the train after the brakes were applied?
a) 1.88m/s²
b) 1.92m/s²
c) 1.96m/s²
d) 2.00m/s²

8. In the above problem, was the driver able to prevent the accident?
a) Yes
b) No
c) Can't be determined
d) None of the above

9. **Acceleration of a moving body can be determined by:**
a) Slope of velocity-time graph
b) Area under velocity time graph
c) Slope of distance time graph
d) Area under distance-time graph

10. **Ratio of the distance travelled by a free falling body in the 1st 3 seconds is:**
a) 1:4:8
b) 1:2:3
c) 1:7:11
d) 1:4:9

11. **Which type of simple machine is used in each case?**
   - Woodcutter using an axe
   - Lady withdrawing water from well
   - Children playing on see-saw
   - A mechanic working with nuts and bolts
a) Screw, Wedge, Pulley, Lever
b) Wedge, Pulley, Lever, Screw
c) Pulley, Lever, Screw, Wedge
d) Lever, Screw, Wedge, Pulley

12. **Which of the following statements is true:**
a) IMA is always > AMA
b) IMA is always < AMA
c) IMA is always = AMA
d) None of the above

13. **Which of the following statements is true:**
   i. F_E is in the middle of the 3rd class lever
   ii. Fulcrum is in the middle of the 1st class lever
   iii. F_R is in the middle of the 2nd class lever
a) Only statement (i) & (ii) are correct
b) All statements are correct
c) Only statement (ii) is correct
d) None of the statements are correct

14. **Consider the following statements:**
   i. Only order 1 and order 2 levers multiply force
   ii. Mechanical Advantage of 3rd order lever is always < 1
a) Statement (i) is true but statement (ii) is false
b) Statement (i) is false but statement (ii) is true
c) Both statements are true, but statement (ii) is not the correct explanation of statement (i)
d) Both statements are true & statement (ii) is the correct explanation of statement (i)

15. In wrestling matches, soft ground is provided instead of hard ground because:

a) During fall, frictional force can cause burns to wrestler

b) Hitting ground is an impulsive force

c) Soft ground provides better recoil

d) None of the above

16. A 100kg stone and a bird feather are allowed to free fall in the vacuum from a height of 50m. The time taken by 100kg stone to reach ground is:

a) Less than the time taken by the feather

b) Greater than the time taken by the feather

c) Equal to the time taken by the feather

d) Infinite as there is no force exerted because the medium is vacuum

Physics Practice Test #1 – ANSWER KEY

1. **Ans. (a)**

   $s = ut + 1/2at2$

   $s = 0*1/2 + 1/2*F/m*8*8$

   $s = 32*5/10 = 16m$

   $W = F \times s = 5 \times 16 = 80 J$

2. **Ans. (b)**

   As the height of an object increases, more P.E. is stored in it. Hence, point B has the highest P.E. Point D has the same mass as point B, same gravitational pull as both are in the same environment and it's lifted to the same height as B. Thus, according to the formula of P.E = mgh both D and B will possess the same potential energy.

3. **Ans. (d)**

   T.E. of the disc = Rotational K.E. + Linear K.E.

   i.e. T.E. = $1/2w2I + 1/2mv2$

   Now, I = $1/2mr2$[BH10] & $v = rw$

   Therefore, T.E. = $1/2*1/2mr2w2 + 1/2mr2w2 = 3/4mr2w2$

4. **Ans. (a)**

   MA of a wedge = L/B

5. **Ans. (c)**

   $a = g(M - m)/(M + m)$

   $a = 9.8(100 - 40)/(100 + 40)$

   $a = 9.8*60/140 = 4.2m/s2$

6. **Ans. (a)**

   Negative for A and positive for B, because both start from rest then A moves downward and B moves going upward.

7. **Ans. (c)**

   $F = umg$

   $F = ma$

   $a = ug = 0.2 \times 9.8 = 1.96m/s2$

8. **Ans. (a)**

   Calculate the distance after which train came to a halt

   $v2 = u2 - 2as$ (as a is deceleration)

   $0 = 302 - 2*1.96*s$

   $s = 900/3.92 = 229.59m$

   This is clearly less than 250m.

9. **Ans. (a)**

    The slope of the velocity time graph gives the acceleration of a moving body.

    The slope of the distance time graph gives the velocity of a moving body.

    Area under velocity time graph gives the displacement of the body.

    Area under distance time graph is not defined in Physics.

10. **Ans. (d)**

    The graph of acceleration is exponential in nature. Therefore:

    Acceleration due to gravity in 1st sec of free fall: $(1)^2 \times 9.8$

    Acceleration due to gravity in 2nd sec of free fall: $(2)^2 \times 9.8$

    Acceleration due to gravity in 3rd sec of free fall: $(3)^2 \times 9.8$

    $= 1 \times 9.8 : 4 \times 9.8 : 9 \times 9.8$

    Cancelling common factor 9.8

    Answer: 1:4:9

11. **Ans. (b)**

    An axe is an example of a wedge.

    Lady is using a pulley with her being on one end of the rope and the bucket of water on another to withdraw water from the well.

    See-saw is an example of 1st order lever.

    Nuts and Bolts fall under the category of screws

12. **Ans. (a)**

    Actual mechanical advantage is always less than (even if slightly) from ideal MA due to friction.

13. **Ans. (b)**

    Remember the various orders/types/classes of levers. All the above statements are true.

    1st class lever has load on one end, effort on another end and fulcrum in the centre.

    2nd class lever load in the middle, effort on one end and fulcrum on the other end.

    3rd class lever has load on the one end, effort in the middle and fulcrum on the other end.

14. **Ans. (d)**

    Mechanical advantage of a lever is given by: length of effort arm/ length of load arm

    M.A. of a 3rd order lever is always less than 1 as the effort arm is smaller than the load arm, whereas in both 1st and 2nd class levers, the effort arm is longer than the load arm.

15. **Ans. (b)**

    Impulse is defined as a large amount of force applied in a very short duration of time. Hence hitting the ground is a type of impulsive force and if the ground is hard, the reactive force is more and the wrestler can get seriously injured.

16. **Ans. (c)**

    All objects free fall at the same rate in the absence of air. The air resistance is responsible for slowing down objects of lighter mass such as feather. But in this case, as the medium is vacuum, both objects will reach ground at the same time.

PRACTICE TEST #2

MATHEMATICS PRACTICE TEST #2

1. $3 * (2 * 4^3) \div 4 =$

2. $(4^3 + 2 - 1) =$

3. What will it cost to carpet a room with indoor/outdoor carpet if the room is 10 feet wide and 12 feet long? The carpet costs $12.51 per square yard.

    a) $166.80.
    b) $175.90.
    c) $184.30.
    d) $189.90.
    e) $192.20.

4. Sally has three pieces of material. The first piece is 1 yard, 2 feet, and 6 inches long; the second piece is 2 yard, 1 foot, and 5 inches long; and the third piece is 4 yards, 2 feet, and 8 inches long. How much material does Sally have?

    a) 7 yards, 1 foot, and 8 inches.
    b) 8 yards, 4 feet, and 4 inches.
    c) 8 yards and 11 inches.
    d) 9 yards and 7 inches.
    e) 10 yards.

5. A vitamin's expiration date has passed. It was supposed to contain 500 mg of Calcium, but it has lost 325 mg of Calcium. How many mg of Calcium are left?

    a) 135 mg.
    b) 175 mg.
    c) 185 mg.
    d) 200 mg.
    e) 220 mg.

6. Jim works for $15.50 per hour at a health care facility. He is supposed to get a $0.75 per hour raise after one year of service. What will be his percent increase in hourly pay?

    a) 2.7%.
    b) 3.3%.
    c) 133%.
    d) 4.8%.
    e) 105%.

7. Edmond has to sell his BMW. He bought the car for $49,000, but sold it at 20% less. At what price did Edmond sell the car?

    a) $24,200.
    b) $28,900.
    c) $35,600.
    d) $37,300.
    e) $39,200.

8. Sarah needs to make a cake and some cookies. The cake requires 3/8 cup of sugar, and the cookies require 3/5 cup of sugar. Sarah has 15/16 cups of sugar. Does she have enough sugar, or how much more does she need?

    a) She has enough sugar.
    b) She needs 1/8 of a cup of sugar.
    c) She needs 3/80 of a cup of sugar.
    d) She needs 4/19 of a cup of sugar.
    e) She needs 1/9 of a cup of sugar.

9. What is the least common multiple of 2, 3, 4, and 5?

    a) 30
    b) 60
    c) 120
    d) 40
    e) 50

10. $\dfrac{3}{4} * \dfrac{4}{5} * \dfrac{5}{3} =$ _____

11. What is the result of multiplication of
$$\frac{100}{30} * \frac{3}{6} * \frac{300}{50}$$

12. $\dfrac{2}{3} + \dfrac{4}{5} - \dfrac{5}{6} =$ _____

13. $\frac{11}{22} + \frac{22}{44} + \frac{1}{2} =$ _____

14. $\frac{13}{4} + \frac{5}{8} =$ _____

15. David had 12 chocolates which he decided to distribute among his friends. Alex got $\frac{2}{3}$ of the total chocolates. How many chocolates did he get?

    a) 2
    b) 4
    c) 8
    d) 9

16. Convert the following to Roman numerals: 240

    a) CCL
    b) DXL
    c) CCXXX
    d) CCXL
    e) None of the above

17. Convert the following into decimal form: $2\frac{1}{2} - 1\frac{1}{4}$

    a) 1.5
    b) 2.25
    c) 1.25
    d) 0.25
    e) 0.75

18. Convert 0.55 into a fraction.

    a) 11/20
    b) 5/9
    c) 5/10
    d) 11/50
    e) 10/20

19. Convert $\frac{7}{20}$ into a decimal form.

    a) 0.45
    b) 0.35
    c) 0.28
    d) 0.65
    e) 0.12

20. If Sam can move a stack of bricks *b* minutes, how many pages can he move in 8 minutes?

    a) 8/*b*.

    b) *b* – 8.

    c) *b* + 8.

    d) *b*/8.

21. A used car is on sale for $2,600, which is a 20% discount off the regular price. Calculate the original price of the used car.

    a) $2800.

    b) $2900.

    c) $3250.

    d) $3560.

22. An amusement park added a 0.5% convenience fee for all ticket purchases. If a visitor to the park spends $40 per ticket, how much will the convenience fee add to the $40 purchase price?

    a) 18 cents.

    b) 12 cents.

    c) 14 cents.

    d) 20 cents.

23. You need to purchase a textbook for nursing school. The book costs $90.00, and the sales tax is 7.25%. You have $100. How much change will you receive back?

    a) $96.53.

    b) $4.47.

    c) $3.47

    d) $6.53.

24. 45% of what number is 90?

    a) 100

    b) 110

    c) 150

    d) 200

25. 5.86 + 1.27 =

    a) 9.13

    b) 7.13

    c) 7.23

    d) 8.13

26. Convert 0.90 to a fraction.
- a) 15/20
- b) 18/20
- c) 7/9
- d) 14/25

27. $6.01 + 11.75 =$
- a) 17.76
- b) 18.78
- c) 16.74
- d) 17.74

28. How many centimeters in one 1.5 kilometers?
- a) 15,000
- b) 1,500.
- c) 100.50
- d) 150,000.

29. $18.75 + 5.17 + 5.37 =$
- a) 8.29
- b) 39.28
- c) 29.29 (correct)
- d) 24.36

30. What is the decimal form of 11/20?
- a) 0.3
- b) 0.55
- c) 0.4
- d) 0.45

31. $22.22 - 11.11 - 2.37 =$
- a) 11.22
- b) 8.74
- c) 7.84
- d) 9.74

32. $4.22 - 2.42 =$
- a) 2.8
- b) 1.8
- c) 3.8
- d) 1.6

33. 5.82 − 4.83 =
    a) 0.99
    b) 1.99
    c) 0.91
    d) 1.09

34. How many millimeters in 1.27 meters?
    a) 1,270
    b) 127
    c) 12,700
    d) 120.7

35. 99 * 0.37 =
    a) 36.63
    b) 37.36
    c) 42.27
    d) 41.83

36. 7.52 * 3 =
    a) 21.25
    b) 22.56
    c) 23.22
    d) 23.51

37. How many milligrams are in a 3grams?
    a) 30,000
    b) 3,000
    c) 300
    d) 1,000

38. Convert 0.55 to a fraction
    a) 11/20
    b) 7/10
    c) 7/9
    d) 11/30

39. What number is 11% of 2000?
    a) 50
    b) 100
    c) 150
    d) 220

40. If a shift is 1100 to 2300 hours, what time does the shift start?

    a) 1:50 am.

    b) 11:00 pm.

    c) 3:00 pm.

    d) 11:00 am.

41. How is 9:45 pm, expressed in military time?

    a) 1545

    b) 1745

    c) 2145

    d) 1945

42. $\frac{12}{8} + \frac{3}{8} =$

    a) $1\frac{5}{8}$

    b) $\frac{5}{49}$

    c) $1\frac{7}{8}$

    d) $1\frac{7}{16}$

43. $\frac{3}{5} \div \frac{2}{10} =$

    a) 3

    b) 3/5

    c) 6

    d) 2.5

44. $\dfrac{6}{7} * \dfrac{3}{7} =$

    a) $\dfrac{9}{7}$

    b) $\dfrac{18}{49}$

    c) $\dfrac{7}{42}$

    d) $\dfrac{9}{49}$

45. What is decimal form of 9/45?
    a) 0.2
    b) 0.7
    c) 0.3
    d) 0.24

46. What is the decimal form of 5/8?
    a) 0.875
    b) 0.755
    c) 0.625
    d) 0.450

47. 27.22 + 9.95 =
    a) 37.17
    b) 33.56
    c) 17.27
    d) 33.65

48. What is the decimal form of 6/15?
    a) 0.3
    b) 0.2
    c) 0.25
    d) 0.4

49. Convert 0.375 to a fraction.
   a) 4/7
   b) 3/8
   c) 5/8
   d) 3/10

50. How many grams are in a 1.25 kilograms?
   a) 125
   b) 250
   c) 1,250
   d) 12,500

Math Practice Test #2 – ANSWER KEY

1. **Answer: 96**

   Explanation: We need to remember the order of operations (PEMDAS) to solve this question. First of all, we solve the parenthesis, and then the exponents. In this particular question, 4^3 is within the parenthesis so we solve it first. $4^3 = 64$. Now, multiplying it with 2 to solve the parenthesis, it becomes $64*2 = 128$. So, the expression becomes $3*128÷4$. Following PEMDAS, we multiply 128 by 3, and then divide the answer by 4. This gives us $384÷4 = 96$

2. **Answer: 65**

   Explanation: We need to remember the order of operations (PEMDAS) to solve this question. First of all, we solve the parenthesis, and then the exponents. In this particular question, 4^3 is within the parenthesis so we solve it first. $4^3 = 64$. Now, the expression becomes (64+2-1). So, we add 2 in 64 first, and then subtract 1 from the answer. This gives us $66-1 = 5$.

3. a) **Explanation:** It is important to note that the rate of the carpet is given is per sq. yard and the dimensions of the room are given in feet. So, we need to convert the width and length of the room in yards, and then calculate the total area of the room. We know that
   1 foot = 0.33 yards
   10 feet = 3.33 yards
   12 feet = 4 yards
   Area of the room = 4*3.33 = 13.32 sq yards
   So, the total cost to carpet this room equals 13.32 * 12.51 ➜ $166.6

4. d) **Explanation:** First of all, we add the inches, feet and yards individually.
   Inches: 6 + 5+ 8 = 19 inches
   Feet = 2 + 1 + 2 = 5 Feet
   Yards = 1 + 2 + 4 = 7 yards

   As we know that there are 12 inches in 1 foot, so 19 inches becomes 1 foot and 7 inches. Therefore, we add one more to 5 feet, which makes it 6 feet.
   Also, we know that 1 foot = 0.33 yards, so 6 feet = 2 yards.

   This makes the total length equal to 9 yards and 7 inches. [9 yards because 7 yards calculated in the first step plus 2 yards from 6 feet conversion to yards.]

5. **b)** **Explanation:** The amount of calcium actually required was 500 mg in that vitamin, but it has lost 325mg of calcium in it. Therefore, it has got 500-325 = 175 mg calcium left in it after expiration.

6. **d)** **Explanation:** His new hourly salary would become $15.50+$0.75 = $16.25

Percentage change = $\frac{Final\ value - Original\ Value}{Original\ Value} * 100$

$\frac{16.25-15.50}{15.50} * 100$

$\frac{0.75}{15.50} * 100 = 4.8\%$

7. **e)** **Explanation:** Price of Edmond's car was $49000 but he had to sell it at 20% less. This means that the price at which he sold his car was 80% of the actual price. Therefore,
0.8*49000 = $39200

8. **c)** **Explanation:** Cake requires $\frac{3}{8} = 0.375$ cup of sugar, whereas, cookies require $\frac{3}{5} = 0.6$ cup of sugar. This makes a total of 0.375+0.6 = 0.975 cup of sugar.

Sarah has got $\frac{15}{16} = 0.9375$ cup of sugar.

Therefore, it is clear that Sarah needs more sugar than she already has got. The exact amount of sugar required can be calculated by subtracting total sugar from required sugar.

i.e. 0.975-0.9375 = 0.0375

Therefore, Option (c) is correct. $[\frac{3}{80} = 0.0375]$

9. **Answer: Option (b)**

Find all the prime numbers that multiply to give the numbers.

For 2, prime factor is 2; for 3, prime factor is 3; for 4, prime factors are 2, 2; for 5, prime factor is 5. Note the maximum times of occurrence of each prime and multiply these to find the least common multiple. The LCM is 2 * 2 * 3 * 5 = 60.

10. Correct Answer: 1

Explanation: If we observe closely, we note that for every number in the numerator, there is an equivalent denominator which cancels the numerator. Therefore the net result of this multiplication comes out to be 1.

11. Answer: 10

Explanation: As explained in the previous questions, you need to look for the numbers which can be cancelled with each other in numerator and denominator. Observing closely, we see that $\frac{300}{30} = 10$. Also, $\frac{100}{50} = 2$, and $\frac{3}{6} = \frac{1}{2}$.

So, $\frac{1}{2} * 10 * 2 = 10$

12. Answer: $\frac{19}{30}$

Explanation: In this question, we find the sum of the given fractions first, and then subtract $\frac{5}{6}$ from that sum.

$\frac{2}{3} + \frac{4}{5}$ ➔ $\frac{10+12}{15} = \frac{22}{15}$

Now, subtracting $\frac{5}{6}$ from it, we get;

$\frac{22}{15} - \frac{5}{6}$ ➔ $\frac{22(6)-5(15)}{90}$ ➔ $\frac{19}{30}$

13. Answer: $\frac{3}{2}$

Explanation: We know that $\frac{11}{22}$ can be written as $\frac{1}{2}$. Similarly, $\frac{22}{44}$ equals $\frac{1}{2}$. Therefore, the expression becomes,

$\frac{1}{2} + \frac{1}{2} + \frac{1}{2}$ ➔ $\frac{3}{2}$

14. Answer: $\frac{31}{8}$

Explanation: This is a relatively simple question. Adding the given fractions, we get;

$\frac{13}{4} + \frac{5}{8}$ ➔ $\frac{13(2)+5}{8}$ ➔ $\frac{26+5}{8}$ ➔ $\frac{31}{8}$

15. Answer: Option (c)

Explanation: $\frac{2}{3}$ of the actual number of chocolates means that Alex got;

$12 * \frac{2}{3} = 4*2$ ➔ 8 Chocolates.

16. Answer: Option (d)

Explanation: CCXL (correct; C = 100, X = 10, L =50. Since X is before L and X is a smaller value than L, it means that you subtract instead of add. So you could visualize it as $100 + 100 - 10 + 50 = 240$. This avoids having to write XXXX to equal 40.)

17. Answer: Option (c)

Explanation: Answer is 1.25

$2.5 - 1.25 = 1.25$

18. Answer: Option (a)

Explanation: Answer is 11/20

0.55 equals 55/100. The lowest common denominator or 55/100 is 5.

$55/5 = 11$ & $100/5 = 20$.

19. Answer: Option (b)

Explanation:

```
        .35  R 0
   20)7.00
      -60
      ____
      100
     -100
      ____
        0
```


20. a) Explanation: From the given information in the question, Sam moves a stack of bricks in 'b' minutes. Now, we are asked about the number of stacks he can move in 8 minutes. The simplest way to solve this question is by writing it in ratio form I.e.

1 stack → 'b' minutes

X stacks → 8 minutes

Cross multiplying the above equations, we get $8*1 = x*b$

Therefore, $x = 8/b$ (Which means that he can move 8/b stacks in 8 minutes)

21. c) Explanation: From the statement of the question, it is clear that when we take 20% off the price of car, it costs $2600. This means that $2600 equals 80% of the actual price of the computer. Writing this in form of an equation;

$0.8 * x = \$2600$

$x = 2600/0.8$

$x = \$3250$ where 'x' is the actual price of the car.

22. d) Explanation: The convenience fee is 5%, i.e. 0.5/100 = 0.005. Multiplying it with $40 gives us the amount of tax amount which hotel has charged to this traveler.
$40* 0.005 = $0.20
Note that the given answer choices are in cents and our answer is in dollars. We convert our answer in to cents by multiplying it with 100. It becomes 20 cents.

23. c) Explanation: This is a tricky question. We are given with the sales tax percentage and the actual amount of the book. First of all, we need to find out the amount we would be charged for this including sales tax, and then we need to subtract it from 100, to find out the change we will receive from them.
7.25% tax on $90 becomes 0.0725*90 = $6.525
So, the total amount that we will be charged becomes 90+ 6.53 = $96.53
Subtracting it from $100 to find the change, we get 100 – 96.53 = $3.47

24. Answer: Option (d) 200
25. Answer: Option (b) 7.13
26. Answer: Option (b) 18/20
27. Answer: Option (a) 17.76
28. Answer: Option (d) 150,000
29. Answer: Option (c) 29.29
30. Answer: Option (b) 0.55
31. Answer: Option (b) 8.74
32. Answer: Option (b) 1.8
33. Answer: Option (a) 0.99
34. Answer: Option (a) 1,270
35. Answer: Option (a) 36.63
36. Answer: Option (b) 22.56
37. Answer: Option (b) 3,000
38. Answer: Option (a) 11/20
39. Answer: Option (d) 220
40. Answer: Option (d) 11:00am

41. Answer: Option (c) 2145

42. Answer: Option (c) $1\frac{7}{8}$

43. Answer: Option (a) 3

44. Answer: Option (b) $\frac{18}{49}$

45. Answer: Option (a) 0.2

46. Answer: Option (c) 0.625

47. Answer: Option (a) 37.17

48. Answer: Option (d) 0.4

49. Answer: Option (b) 3/8

50. Answer: Option (c) 1,250

READING SECTION PRACTICE TEST #2

I don't know whether you have ever seen a map of a person's mind. Doctors sometimes draw maps of other parts of you, and your own map can become intensely interesting, but catch them trying to draw a map of a child's mind, which is not only confused, but keeps going round all the time. There are zigzag lines on it, just like your temperature on a card, and these are probably roads in the island, for the Neverland is always more or less an island, with astonishing splashes of color here and there, and coral reefs and rakish-looking craft in the offing, and savages and lonely lairs, and gnomes who are mostly tailors, and caves through which a river runs, and princes with six elder brothers, and a hut fast going to decay, and one very small old lady with a hooked nose. It would be an easy map if that were all, but there is also first day at school, religion, fathers, the round pond, needle-work, murders, hangings, verbs that take the dative, chocolate pudding day, getting into braces, say ninety-nine, three-pence for pulling out your tooth yourself, and so on, and either these are part of the island or they are another map showing through, and it is all rather confusing, especially as nothing will stand still.

1. What is the main idea of the passage?
    a. Children's minds are simpler than adult minds.
    b. Children's minds are more complex than adult minds.
    c. No one can map the human mind.
    d. Doctors can map children's minds.

2. Which statement is not a detail from the passage?
    a. Peter Pan lives in Neverland.
    b. Neverland is more or less an island.
    c. Gnomes are mostly tailors.
    d. There is chocolate pudding day.

3. What is the meaning of <u>rakish</u> in the middle of the paragraph?
    a. Zigzag
    b. Sailing
    c. Sinking
    d. Streamlined

4. What is the author's primary purpose in writing this passage?
    a. To entertain young readers
    b. To entertain adult readers
    c. To educate children about Neverland
    d. To explain the existence of Neverland

5. Which is the best summary of this passage?
    a. Children's minds are jumbled and confusing.
    b. Adult minds are jumbled and confusing.
    c. Children think about mundane things.
    d. Children are imaginative.

The situation of the house was good. High hills rose immediately behind, and at no great distance on each side; some of which were open downs, the others cultivated and woody. The village of Barton was chiefly on one of these hills, and formed a pleasant view from the cottage windows. The prospect in front was more extensive; it commanded the whole of the valley, and reached into the country beyond. The hills which surrounded the cottage terminated the valley in that direction; under another name, and in another course, it branched out again between two of the steepest of them.

With the size and furniture of the house Mrs. Dashwood was upon the whole well satisfied; for though her former style of life rendered many additions to the latter indispensable, yet to add and improve was a delight to her; and she had at this time ready money enough to supply all that was wanted of greater elegance to the apartments. "As for the house itself, to be sure," said she, "it is too small for our family, but we will make ourselves tolerably comfortable for the present, as it is too late in the year for improvements. Perhaps in the spring, if I have plenty of money, as I dare say I shall, we may think about building. These parlors are both too small for such parties of our friends as I hope to see often collected here; and I have some thoughts of throwing the passage into one of them with perhaps a part of the other, and so leave the remainder of that other for an entrance; this, with a new drawing room which may be easily added, and a bed-chamber and garret above, will make it a very snug little cottage. I could wish the stairs were handsome. But one must not expect everything; though, I suppose it would be no difficult matter to widen them. I shall see how much I am before-hand with the world in the spring, and we will plan our improvements accordingly."

6. What is the main idea of the passage?
    a. The house is well-placed.
    b. The house is too small.
    c. The house could be improved.
    d. The house is quite poor.

7. Which statement is not a detail from the passage?
    a. The parlors are too small.
    b. There is a garret above the drawing room.
    c. The cottage has hills behind it.
    d. Mrs. Dashwood has nice furnishings.

8. What is the meaning of <u>indispensable</u> in the second paragraph?
    a. Necessary
    b. Unnecessary
    c. Unappealing
    d. Appealing

9. What is the author's primary purpose in writing this passage?
    a. To create a visual impression of the house
    b. To provide insights into Mrs. Dashwood's character
    c. To show how Mrs. Dashwood felt about the cottage
    d. To illustrate Mrs. Dashwood's financial state

10. Which is the best summary of this passage?
    a. Mrs. Dashwood finds the cottage lovely, but inadequate.
    b. Mrs. Dashwood would like a smaller home.
    c. Mrs. Dashwood is quite wealthy.
    d. Mrs. Dashwood is impoverished.

The division of the world being now satisfactorily arranged, it would seem that all things ought to have gone on smoothly, but such was not the case. Trouble arose in an unlooked-for quarter. The Giants, those hideous monsters (some with legs formed of serpents) who had sprung from the earth and the blood of Uranus, declared war against the triumphant deities of Olympus, and a struggle ensued, which, in consequence of Gæa having made these children of hers invincible as long as they kept their feet on the ground, was wearisome and protracted. Their mother's precaution, however, was rendered unavailing by pieces of rock being hurled upon them, which threw them down, and their feet being no longer placed firmly on their mother-earth, they were overcome, and this tedious war (which was called the Gigantomachia) at last came to an end. Among the most daring of these earth-born giants were Enceladus, Rhœtus, and the valiant Mimas, who, with youthful fire and energy, hurled against heaven great masses of rock and burning oak-trees, and defied the lightning of Zeus. One of the most powerful monsters who opposed Zeus in this war was called Typhon or Typhœus. He was the youngest son of Tartarus and Gæa, and had a hundred heads, with eyes which struck terror to the beholders, and awe-inspiring voices frightful to hear. This dreadful monster resolved to conquer both gods and men, but his plans were at length defeated by Zeus, who, after a violent encounter, succeeded in destroying him with a thunderbolt, but not before he had so terrified the gods that they had fled for refuge to Egypt, where they metamorphosed themselves into different animals and thus escaped.

11. What is the main idea of the passage?
    a. Zeus had to fight the Giants
    b. Gaea was the mother of the gods.
    c. Gaea was the mother of the Giants.
    d. The Giants won the battle.

12. Which statement is not a detail from the passage?
    a. Zeus was called Typhon
    b. Zeus was the son of Gaea
    c. Zeus was the husband of Hera
    d. Zeus was the son of Tartarus

13. What is the meaning of triumphant in the paragraph?
    a. Failing
    b. Greek
    c. Victorious
    d. Immoral

14. What is the author's primary purpose in writing this passage?
    a. To entertain the reader
    b. To share stories from mythology
    c. To provide religious education
    d. To show why Greek mythology is wrong

15. Which is the best summary of this passage?
    a. The Giants were monstrous and evil.
    b. The Greek gods of Olympus had to defeat the Giants.
    c. The Giants are the precursors of the gods.
    d. Greek mythology is violent.

"Oh, I can carry it," the child responded cheerfully. "It isn't heavy. I've got all my worldly goods in it, but it isn't heavy. And if it isn't carried in just a certain way the handle pulls out—so I'd better keep it because I know the exact knack of it. It's an extremely old carpet-bag. Oh, I'm very glad you've come, even if it would have been nice to sleep in a wild cherry-tree. We've got to drive a long piece, haven't we? Mrs. Spencer said it was eight miles. I'm glad because I love driving. Oh, it seems so wonderful that I'm going to live with you and belong to you. I've never belonged to anybody—not really. But the asylum was the worst. I've only been in it four months, but that was enough. I don't suppose you ever were an orphan in an asylum, so you can't possibly understand what it is like. It's worse than anything you could imagine. Mrs. Spencer said it was wicked of me to talk like that, but I didn't mean to be wicked. It's so easy to be wicked without knowing it, isn't it? They were good, you know—the asylum people. But there is so little scope for the imagination in an asylum—only just in the other orphans. It was pretty interesting to imagine things about them— to imagine that perhaps the girl who sat next to you was really the daughter of a belted earl, who had been stolen away from her parents in her infancy by a cruel nurse who died before she could confess. I used to lie awake at nights and imagine things like that, because I didn't have time in the day. I guess that's why I'm so thin—I AM dreadful thin, ain't I? There isn't a pick on my bones. I do love to imagine I'm nice and plump, with dimples in my elbows."

16. What is the main idea of the passage?
    a. The girl is an orphan.
    b. The girl has been in an orphanage.
    c. The girl is excited and imaginative.
    d. The girl in the orphanage is the daughter of an earl.

17. Which statement is not a detail from the passage?
    a. The child has an old carpet-bag.
    b. The child loves driving.
    c. The child is thin.
    d. The asylum was a horrible place.

18. What is the meaning of asylum in the paragraph?
    a. Hospital
    b. Sanitarium
    c. Orphanage
    d. Prison

19. What is the author's primary purpose in writing this passage?
    a. To illustrate the child's excitement.
    b. To educate the reader.
    c. To explain why orphanages were bad.
    d. To create the setting.

20. Which is the best summary of this passage?
    a. The child is frightened of the changes in her life.
    b. The child is excited by the changes in her life.
    c. The family is unhappy about the child.
    d. The family is happy about the child.

For my own part, I had been feverishly excited all day. Something very like the war fever that occasionally runs through a civilized community had got into my blood, and in my heart I was not so very sorry that I had to return to Maybury that night. I was even afraid that that last fusillade I had heard might mean the extermination of our invaders from Mars. I can best express my state of mind by saying that I wanted to be in at the death.

It was nearly eleven when I started to return. The night was unexpectedly dark; to me, walking out of the lighted passage of my cousins' house, it seemed indeed black, and it was as hot and close as the day. Overhead the clouds were driving fast, albeit not a breath stirred the shrubs about us. My cousins' man lit both lamps. Happily, I knew the road intimately. My wife stood in the light of the doorway, and watched me until I jumped up into the dog cart. Then abruptly she turned and went in, leaving my cousins side by side wishing me good hap.

I was a little depressed at first with the contagion of my wife's fears, but very soon my thoughts reverted to the Martians. At that time I was absolutely in the dark as to the course of the evening's fighting. I did not know even the circumstances that had precipitated the conflict. As I came through Ockham (for that was the way I returned, and not through Send and Old Woking) I saw along the western horizon a blood-red glow, which as I drew nearer, crept slowly up the sky. The driving clouds of the gathering thunderstorm mingled there with masses of black and red smoke.

21. What is the main idea of the passage?
    a. Martians are going to invade.
    b. The man is fighting the Martians.
    c. The Martians caused a thunderstorm.
    d. The narrator is traveling at a time when Martians had invaded.

22. Which statement is not a detail from the passage?
    a. He is leaving his cousins' home.
    b. Humans had fought the Martians all evening.
    c. He travelled through Send.
    d. He travelled through Ockham.

23. What is the meaning of <u>fusillade</u> in the first paragraph?
    a. Battle
    b. Series of shots
    c. Trains
    d. Spaceship

24. What is the author's primary purpose in writing this passage?
    a. To educate
    b. To tell a story
    c. To create a character
    d. To create the setting

25. Which is the best summary of this passage?
    a. The narrator is fighting the Martians.
    b. Martians have destroyed Ockham.
    c. The narrator wants to fight the Martians.
    d. The Martians have won the battle for earth.

What I felt the next day was, I suppose, nothing that could be fairly called a reaction from the cheer of my arrival; it was probably at the most only a slight oppression produced by a fuller measure of the scale, as I walked round them, gazed up at them, took them in, of my new circumstances. They had, as it were, an extent and mass for which I had not been prepared and in the presence of which I found myself, freshly, a little scared as well as a little proud. Lessons, in this agitation, certainly suffered some delay; I reflected that my first duty was, by the gentlest arts I could contrive, to win the child into the sense of knowing me. I spent the day with her out-of-doors; I arranged with her, to her great satisfaction, that it should be she, she only, who might show me the place. She showed it step by step and room by room and secret by secret, with droll, delightful, childish talk about it and with the result, in half an hour, of our becoming immense friends. Young as she was, I was struck, throughout our little tour, with her confidence and courage with the way, in empty chambers and dull corridors, on crooked staircases that made me pause and even on the summit of an old machicolated square tower that made me dizzy, her morning music, her disposition to tell me so many more things than she asked, rang out and led me on.

26. What is the main idea of the passage?
    a. The narrator wants to get to know the child.
    b. The child is ill-behaved.
    c. The narrator does not like the child.
    d. The child lives in a big house.

27. Which statement is not a detail from the passage?
    a. The child showed him the house.
    b. The house has a square tower.
    c. His first duty was to get to know the child.
    d. They began lessons that day.

28. What is the meaning of agitation in the paragraph?
    a. A state of anxiety
    b. A state of anger
    c. A state of excitement
    d. A state of happiness

29. What is the author's primary purpose in writing this passage?
   a. To educate the reader about nannies.
   b. To illustrate the child's character.
   c. To show the relationship between the caregiver and child.
   d. To show the relationship between the parent and child.

30. Which is the best summary of this passage?
   a. The narrator is a caregiver, who has met a young charge for the first time.
   b. The narrator is a parent caring for her child.
   c. The child is an orphan, newly adopted.
   d. The house is in poor repair.

One is always profoundly impressed by the expression of a sense of bulk, vastness, or mass in form. There is a feeling of being lifted out of one's puny self to something bigger and more stable. It is this splendid feeling of bigness in Michael Angelo's figures that is so satisfying. One cannot come away from the contemplation of that wonderful ceiling of his in the Vatican without the sense of having experienced something of a larger life than one had known before. Never has the dignity of man reached so high an expression in paint, a height that has been the despair of all who have since tried to follow that lonely master. In landscape also this expression of largeness is fine: one likes to feel the weight and mass of the ground, the vastness of the sky and sea, the bulk of a mountain.
On the other hand one is charmed also by the expression of lightness. This may be noted in much of the work of Botticelli and the Italians of the fifteenth century. Botticelli's figures seldom have any weight; they drift about as if walking on air, giving a delightful feeling of otherworldliness. The hands of the Madonna that hold the Child might be holding flowers for any sense of support they express. It is, I think, on this sense of lightness that a great deal of the exquisite charm of Botticelli's drawing depends.

The feathery lightness of clouds and of draperies blown by the wind is always pleasing, and Botticelli nearly always has a light wind passing through his draperies to give them this sense.

31. What is the main idea of the passage?
   a. Heaviness or bulk is the most impressive quality of a painting.
   b. Both heaviness and lightness can be profoundly impressive.
   c. While heaviness is impressive, lightness is charming.
   d. Lightness is more pleasing than heaviness.

32. Which statement is not a detail from the passage?
   a. Michelangelo creates a feeling of bigness.
   b. Botticelli's paintings are quite light.
   c. The hands of the Madonna hold the Child.
   d. Michelangelo painted a Madonna and Child in the Vatican.

33. What is the meaning of contemplation in the first paragraph?
   a. Examining
   b. Staring
   c. Glancing
   d. Disliking

34. What is the author's primary purpose in writing this passage?
    a. To entertain the reader with descriptions of art.
    b. To explain qualities of Renaissance art.
    c. To show why Renaissance art is the highest quality.
    d. To show why Michelangelo is better than Botticelli.

35. Which is the best summary of this passage?
    a. Both lightness and heaviness can bring appealing qualities to paintings.
    b. Michelangelo's work is quite massive and heavy.
    c. Botticelli's work is light and delicate.
    d. Renaissance paintings are in churches.

Regardless of the time of the year or the time of the day there are pies. The Pennsylvania Dutch eat pies for breakfast. They eat pies for lunch. They eat pies for dinner and they eat pies for midnight snacks. Pies are made with a great variety of ingredients from the apple pie we all know to the rivel pie which is made from flour, sugar, and butter. The Dutch housewife is as generous with her pies as she is with all her cooking, baking six or eight at a time not one and two.

The apple is an important Pennsylvania Dutch food. Dried apples form the basis for many typical dishes. Each fall barrels of apples are converted into cider. Apple butter is one of the Pennsylvania Dutch foods which has found national acceptance. The making of apple butter is an all-day affair and has the air of a holiday to it. Early in the morning the neighbors gather and begin to peel huge piles of apples that will be needed. Soon the great copper apple butter kettle is brought out and set up over a wood fire. Apple butter requires constant stirring to prevent burning. However, stirring can be light work for a boy and a girl when they're young and the day is bright and the world is full of promise. By dusk the apple butter is made, neighborhood news is brought up to date and hunger has been driven that much further away for the coming winter.

Food is abundant and appetites are hearty in the Pennsylvania Dutch country. The traditional dishes are relatively simple and unlike most regional cookery the ingredients are readily available. Best of all, no matter who makes them the results are "wonderful good."

36. What is the main idea of the passage?
    a. Pie is good.
    b. Pennsylvania Dutch housewives cooked a variety of delicious foods.
    c. Apple butter is a Pennsylvania Dutch tradition.
    d. Pies are traditionally Dutch.

37. Which statement is not a detail from the passage?
    a. Pies are made from mincemeat.
    b. Apple butter takes all day.
    c. Traditional Pennsylvania Dutch foods are simple.
    d. The ingredients are widely available.

38. What is the meaning of <u>abundant</u> in the last paragraph?
    a. Scarce
    b. Ample
    c. Free
    d. Inexpensive

39. What is the author's primary purpose in writing this passage?
    a. To explain the history of apple butter
    b. To teach the reader how to make a pie
    c. To introduce Pennsylvania Dutch cooking
    d. To explain how to make an apple pie

40. Which is the best summary of this passage?
    a. Pennsylvania Dutch cooking is simple and "wonderful good".
    b. Pennsylvania Dutch cooking takes all day.
    c. Pennsylvania Dutch people eat a lot of pie.
    d. Everyone should learn to make pie.

Malvern Hill, a plateau a mile and a half long and half a mile wide, with its top bare of woods, commanded a view of the country over which the Confederates must approach. Around the summit of this hill McClellan had placed tier after tier of batteries, arranged like an amphitheater. On the top were placed several heavy siege guns, his left flank being protected by the gunboats in the river. The morning and early afternoon were occupied by several Confederate attacks, sometimes formidable in their nature, but Lee planned for no general move until he could bring up a force which he thought sufficient to attack the strong position of the Federals. The Confederates had orders to advance, when a signal shout was given by the men of Armistead's brigade. The attack was made late in the afternoon by General D. H. Hill, and was gallantly done, but no army could have withstood the fire from the batteries of McClellan as they were massed upon Malvern Hill. All during the evening brigade after brigade tried to force the Union lines. They were forced to breast one of the most devastating storms of lead and canister to which an assaulting army has ever been subjected. The round shot and grape cut through the branches of the trees. Column after column of Southern soldiers rushed upon the death dealing cannon, only to be mowed down. Their thin lines rallied again and again to the charge, but to no avail. McClellan's batteries still hurled their missiles of death. The field below was covered with the dead, as mute pleaders in the cause of peace. The heavy shells from the gunboats on the river shrieked through the timber and great limbs were torn from the trees as they hurtled by. Darkness was falling over the combatants. It was nine o'clock before the guns ceased firing, and only an occasional shot rang out over the gory field of Malvern Hill.

41. What is the main idea of the passage?
    a. The Battle of Malvern Hill was long, drawn out, and bloody.
    b. The Confederates won the Battle of Malvern Hill.
    c. The Union won the Battle of Malvern Hill.
    d. Cannons were used in the Battle.

42. Which statement is not a detail from the passage?
    a. Cannons shot Southern soldiers.
    b. The Union held a high position.
    c. General McClellan commanded the Confederates.
    d. General McClellan commanded the Union troops.

43. What is the meaning of <u>combatants</u> near the end of the paragraph?
    a. Commanders
    b. Soldiers
    c. Dead
    d. Confederates

44. What is the author's primary purpose in writing this passage?
    a. To entertain the reader
    b. To argue with strategies used at Malvern Hill
    c. To educate the reader about the Battle of Malvern Hill
    d. To show the context of the Battle of Malvern Hill

45. Which is the best summary of this passage?
    a. The Battle of Malvern Hill was a decisive Union victory.
    b. The Confederates made poor choices at Malvern Hill.
    c. The Battle of Malvern Hill was an unimportant one.
    d. The Civil War led to many deaths.

Gregory of Tours informs us, that when Frédégonde, wife of Chilpéric, gave the hand of her daughter Rigouthe to the son of the Gothic king, fifty chariots were required to carry away all the valuable objects which composed the princess's dower. A strange family scene, related by the same historian, gives us an idea of the private habits of the court of that terrible queen of the Franks. "The mother and daughter had frequent quarrels, which sometimes ended in the most violent encounters. Frédégonde said one day to Rigouthe, 'Why do you continually trouble me? Here are the goods of your father, take them and do as you like with them.' And conducting her to a room where she locked up her treasures, she opened a large box filled with valuables. After having pulled out a great number of jewels which she gave to her daughter, she said, 'I am tired; put your own hands in the box, and take what you find.' Rigouthe bent down to reach the objects placed at the bottom of the box; upon which Frédégonde immediately lowered the lid on her daughter, and pressed upon it with so much force that the eyes began to start out of the princess's head. A maid began screaming, 'Help! my mistress is being murdered by her mother!' and Rigouthe was saved from an untimely end." It is further related that this was only one of the minor crimes attributed by history to Frédégonde *the Terrible*, who always carried a dagger or poison about with her.

46. What is the main idea of the passage?
    a. The Franks treasured jewels.
    b. Fredegonde was a horrible mother and person.
    c. The Franks had no interest in gold or jewels.
    d. Fredegonde was a good person and queen.

47. Which statement is not a detail from the passage?
    a. Fredegonde tried to kill her daughter.
    b. Fredegonde had a trunk.
    c. A maid saved Fredegonde.
    d. Fredegonde is the daughter's name.

48. What is the meaning of <u>untimely</u> at the end of the paragraph?
    a. Premature
    b. Missed
    c. Late
    d. Forgotten

49. What is the author's primary purpose in writing this passage?
    a. To show how valuable dowries were.
    b. To recount a historical anecdote.
    c. To entertain the reader.
    d. To educate the reader about the facts of early medieval history.

50. Which is the best summary of this passage?
    a. Gregory of Tours was a historian.
    b. Fredegonde was a terrible and murderous person.
    c. Rigouthe had a large dowry.
    d. Jewels were stored in chests.

Reading Practice Test #2 – ANSWER KEY

1. B		26. A	
2. A		27. D	
3. D		28. A	
4. A		29. C	
5. A		30. A	
6. C		31. C	
7. B		32. D	
8. A		33. A	
9. C		34. B	
10. A		35. A	
11. A		36. B	
12. C		37. A	
13. C		38. B	
14. B		39. C	
15. B		40. A	
16. C		41. A	
17. D		42. C	
18. C		43. B	
19. A		44. C	
20. B		45. A	
21. D		46. B	
22. C		47. D	
23. B		48. A	
24. B		49. B	
25. C		50. B	

GRAMMAR PRACTICE TEST #2

1. Select the best word for the blank. _____ to school and study hard to do well in life.
   a. Go
   b. Goes
   c. Going
   d. Gone

2. Which of the following is correct?
   a. Take the dog of the vet.
   b. You need to take the dog to the vet.
   c. The dog need to go to the vet.
   d. The dogs need to going to the vet.

3. Which of the following is grammatically incorrect?
   a. Take the garbage to the curb.
   b. You should take the garbage to the curb.
   c. The garbage needs to go to the curb.
   d. You takes the garbage to the curb.

4. Select the best word for the blank. The hospital cafeteria opens _____ 8:00 AM.
   a. For
   b. At
   c. When
   d. To

5. Which of the following is correct?
   a. The Treaty of Versailles ends World War.
   b. World War I ended with the Treaty of Versailles.
   c. Signed at the end of the war, the treaty surrendered.
   d. The Treaty of Versailles surrender of Germany at the end of the war.

6. Which of the following is grammatically incorrect?
   a. I need to finish reading chapter nine for class tomorrow.
   b. I finish reading chapter nine for class tomorrow.
   c. Tomorrow, I need to finish reading chapter nine for class.
   d. I finished reading chapter nine for tomorrow's class.

7. Select the best word for the blank. When _____ you graduate from nursing school?
   a. Does
   b. Are
   c. Will
   d. Have

8. Which of the following is correct?
   a. It has already been changed.
   b. It already has been changed.
   c. It has been already changed.
   d. Already, it has been changed.

9. Which of the following is grammatically incorrect?
   a. His hobbies include knitting, motorcycle riding, and cooking.
   b. His hobbies include knitting motorcycle riding and cooking.
   c. His hobbies are knitting, motorcycle riding and cooking.
   d. He enjoys knitting, motorcycle riding and cooking.

10. Which of the following is correct?
   a. We have planned a trip to the art museum.
   b. Plan a trips to the art museum.
   c. We plans a trip to the art museum.
   d. The art museum planned a trip.

11. Select the best word for the blank. She often _____ a nap before her shift.
   a. Taken
   b. Took
   c. Takes
   d. Naps

12. Which of the following is correct?
   a. Did you takes his blood pressure?
   b. Do you take his blood pressure?
   c. Did you take his blood pressure?
   d. Did you take him blood pressure?

13. Select the best word for the blank. You will have to buy several _____ of scrubs for work.
   a. Sets
   b. Outfit
   c. Set
   d. Type

14. Which of the following is correct?
   a. Did you pick up the kids from school?
   b. Did you pick the kids from school?
   c. Did you pick up the kids from schools?
   d. Did you pick up the kid to school?

15. Which of the following is grammatically incorrect?
   a. We are planning a summer road trip.
   b. We are planning a road trip this summer.
   c. We are planning a summer vacation.
   d. We are planning a road trip last summer.

16. Select the best word for the blank. Please stop ____ the pharmacy on your way home.
    a. To
    b. From
    c. For
    d. By

17. Which of the following is correct?
    a. Jet lag made it difficult to get up in time for work.
    b. Jet lag make it difficult to get up in time for work.
    c. Jet lag made it difficult to up in time for work.
    d. Jet lag cause difficulty getting up in time for work.

18. Which of the following is grammatically incorrect?
    a. She volunteered at a homeless shelter on the weekends.
    b. She volunteers at a homeless shelter on the weekends.
    c. She will volunteer at a homeless shelter this weekend.
    d. She volunteered at a homeless shelters last weekend.

19. Select the best word for the blank. The patient in room 202 is _____ of a headache.
    a. Complained
    b. Complaining
    c. Complains
    d. Complain

20. Which of the following is grammatically incorrect?
    a. Not all sentences have a direct object.
    b. Not all sentences have a subject.
    c. Not all sentences have a object.
    d. Not all sentences have a predicate adjective.

21. Which word or phrase is the direct object? Take the night off.
    a. Take
    b. Take the night
    c. Night
    d. Night off

22. Which of the following is grammatically incorrect?
    a. The movie was released in October.
    b. The movie will be released in October.
    c. We will release the movie in October.
    d. The movie will release in October.

23. Select the best word for the blank. Nausea ____ common after surgery.
    a. Is
    b. Are
    c. Will
    d. Were

24. Which of the following is grammatically incorrect?
   a. I received a speeding ticket on Highway 72 last week.
   b. I got a speeding ticket on Highway 72 last week.
   c. I was ticketed for speeding on Highway 72 last week.
   d. I was tickets for speeding on Highway 72 last week.

25. Which word or phrase is the direct object? He dresses for dinner every night.
   a. He dresses
   b. Every night
   c. For dinner
   d. Dinner

26. Select the best word for the blank. Saturday night _____ especially chaotic in the emergency room after a large accident.
   a. Is
   b. Are
   c. Were
   d. Was

27. Select the best word for the blank. Drive _____ in the snow to avoid an accidently.
   a. Quickly
   b. Carefully
   c. Carelessly
   d. Recklessly

28. Which word or phrase is the predicate? The little girl plays with a red ball.
   a. The little girl
   b. Girl
   c. Plays
   d. Plays with a red ball.

29. Select the best word for the blank. Where _____ you going to school?
   a. Will
   b. Are
   c. Did
   d. Do

30. Which word or phrase is the predicate? He ran a mile.
   a. He
   b. Ran
   c. He ran
   d. Ran a mile

31. Select the best word for the blank. The doctor, _____ has several specialties, is frequently overbooked.
    a. Which
    b. With
    c. Who
    d. Whom

32. Which word is a noun? Take the kids to school on your way.
    a. Your
    b. Take
    c. Kids
    d. On

33. Which word is a noun? I am making lasagna for dinner on Sunday night.
    a. Lasagna
    b. For
    c. Am
    d. On

34. Which word is a conjunction? He was very busy, yet still made time for volunteer work.
    a. Yet
    b. Still
    c. Was
    d. Time

35. Which word is a conjunction? She wanted to be a doctor, so studied hard.
    a. Wanted
    b. To
    c. Be
    d. So

36. Which word or phrase is a preposition? The books sit on low shelves so they are easy to reach.
    a. So they are easy to reach
    b. The books sit on low shelves
    c. On low shelves
    d. The books sit

37. Which word or phrase is a preposition? She collects dolls and stores them in china cabinets.
    a. She collects
    b. Dolls
    c. Stores them
    d. In china cabinets

38. Which word or phrase is the subject? The book is collecting dust on the shelf, as no one wants to read it.
    a. Shelf
    b. Dust
    c. Book
    d. No one

39. Which word or phrase is the subject? Many people take vitamins to improve their health.
    a. Health
    b. Many
    c. Many people
    d. Vitamins

40. Select the word used incorrectly. She was sleeping in the floor.
    a. She
    b. Was
    c. In
    d. Floor

41. Which is the dependent clause? The children, who have known each other for years, play together very well.
    a. The children
    b. Who have known each other for years
    c. For years
    d. Play together very well

42. Which is the dependent clause? The cats that were for adoption were on display at the pet store.
    a. The cats
    b. Were on display
    c. At the pet store
    d. That were for adoption

43. Select the word used incorrectly. Pick up yours room before company arrives.
    a. Pick
    b. Yours
    c. Company
    d. Before

44. Which has a predicate adjective?
    a. The cat is sleepy.
    b. The cat sleeps in the sun.
    c. The cat slept on the pillow.
    d. The cat likes sunbeams.

45. The following sentence contains which type of phrase? I wanted to go to the movie; however, I have to wait for my sister.
    a. Dependent clause
    b. Conjunction
    c. Contraction
    d. Transitional word

46. The following sentence contains which type of phrase? Please carry the books to the desk in the library.
    a. Conjunction
    b. Transitional word
    c. Prepositional phrase
    d. Predicate adjective

47. Which has a predicate adjective?
    a. The car runs poorly.
    b. I need to wash the car.
    c. Put gas in the car today.
    d. We need to take the car to the repair shop.

48. Select the best substitute for the underlined word. We will be visiting the zoo on Saturday.
    a. Visited
    b. Visit
    c. Plan to visit
    d. Have visited

49. Select the best substitute for the underlined word. I was called into the office early today.
    a. Was phoned
    b. Was summoned
    c. Would be called
    d. Will be called

50. Which of the following is correct?
    a. The pizza was hot, fresh and delicious.
    b. The hot fresh pizza was delicious.
    c. The pizza was hot and fresh delicious.
    d. The pizza has hot, fresh and delicious.

Grammar Practice Test #2 – ANSWER KEY

1. A Go agrees with the implied subject, you.
2. B A has a preposition error, C and D have verb errors.
3. D Subject and verb do not agree.
4. B At refers to time or place.
5. B A has a verb tense issue, C and D don't make sense.
6. B Verb tense does not fit the sentence.
7. C Will is the correct tense, implying ongoing activity.
8. A A is the most correct usage.
9. B B is missing a comma.
10. A The others have errors including subject and verb agreement, confusion of singular and plural and word order.
11. C Present tense takes fits best in the sentence.
12. B Subject/verb agreement is a problem in A & C, while him takes the place of his in D.
13. A Sets is the only plural option.
14. A Prepositions are incorrect in all other options.
15. D Verb tense is incorrect.
16. D By is the correct preposition with "stop".
17. A B and D have verb errors. C is missing a word.
18. D Article and noun do not agree.
19. B Present tense, gerund.
20. C Article and noun do not agree.
21. C Night is the direct object of take.
22. D The movie cannot release itself, so the subject is incorrect.
23. A Verb is agrees with the subject, nausea.
24. D Tickets is a noun, rather than part of a passive verb.
25. D Dinner is the direct object of dresses.
26. D Was agrees with Saturday night.
27. B Carefully is correct, the rest of the words do not fit the sentence.
28. D Everything after the subject, or the little girl, is the predicate.
29. B Are implies the present tense when paired with going.
30. D Ran a mile, or everything after the subject he, is the predicate.
31. C Who is correct. Whom implies a direct object, while with and which don't make sense.
32. C Kids is the only noun, or person, place or thing, listed.
33. A Lasagna is the only noun, or person, place or thing, listed.
34. A Yet is the only conjunction of the words listed.
35. D So is a conjunction, joining parts of the sentence together.
36. C On low shelves identifies place and is a prepositional phrase.
37. D In china cabinets is a prepositional phrase stating where something is.
38. C The book is the subject.
39. C Many people is the subject.
40. C In is incorrect. She would have been sleeping on the floor.
41. B Who have known each other for years is the dependent clause, unable to stand alone in a statement.
42. D That were for adoption is the dependent clause, providing information, but not a statement.
43. B Yours is used incorrectly here.

44. A Sleepy describes the subject, or the cat.
45. D However is a transitional word, showing a contrast between the first part of the sentence and the second.
46. C This sentence has two prepositional phrases, to the desk and in the library.
47. A Poorly describes the car.
48. C Will be visiting and plan to visit both imply a future time.
49. B Call, in this usage, means to summon.
50. A This is the only correct adjective usage. Others are missing commas or have incorrect word order.

VOCABULARY PRACTICE TEST #2

1. Which word is a synonym for <u>slow</u>?
    a. Languid
    b. Fatigued
    c. Immobile
    d. Weary

2. Select the meaning of the underlined word. Do not leave the door to the office <u>ajar</u>.
    a. Closed
    b. Locked
    c. Latched
    d. Open

3. Select the meaning of the underlined word. <u>Terrified</u> of heights, he tried not to look down as he crossed the narrow bridge.
    a. Wary
    b. Fond
    c. Full
    d. Scared

4. What is the best description of the underlined word? She <u>goes</u> to class on Saturdays.
    a. Subject
    b. Verb
    c. Noun
    d. Adverb

5. Select the meaning of the underlined word. It was her turn to <u>supervise</u> the children on the playground.
    a. Teach
    b. Watch
    c. Play with
    d. Release

6. Which word that means <u>looked</u> best fits this sentence? She _____ at the sun setting over the hills.
    a. Stared
    b. Glared
    c. Watched
    d. Gazed

7. Select the word or phrase that is grammatically correct. Because I want to go to bed early tonight, I _____ the dishes now.
    a. Will doing
    b. Am doing
    c. To doing
    d. To do

8. Which of the following sentences is an example of a euphemism?
    a. When the company closed, the employees were let go.
    b. She volunteered at a homeless shelter.
    c. He departed for the airport.
    d. She moved into a new apartment.

9. Which word is not spelled correctly?
    a. Practitioner
    b. Interpreter
    c. Anterior
    d. Lisensed

10. Select the meaning of the underlined word. The lamp <u>illuminated</u> the room with soft, glowing light.
    a. Lit
    b. Warmed
    c. Darkened
    d. Hid

11. Which word that means <u>cleaned</u> best fits this sentence? She carefully _____ her wool sweaters before storing them for the winter.
    a. Scrubbed
    b. Scoured
    c. Laundered
    d. Mopped

12. Which word is a synonym for <u>walked</u>?
    a. Raced
    b. Rushed
    c. Crawled
    d. Strolled

13. Select the meaning of the underlined word. She put away the <u>remainder</u> of her meal for lunch the following day.
    a. Rest
    b. Garbage
    c. Worst
    d. Best

14. What is the best description of the underlined word? She is <u>walking</u> in the park.
    a. Adverb
    b. Gerund
    c. Verb
    d. Adjective

15. Select the meaning of the underlined word. She's a very <u>finicky</u> eater, avoiding most vegetables.
    a. Fast
    b. Slow
    c. Picky
    d. Daring

16. Which word means <u>breathing</u>?
    a. Perspiration
    b. Arrhythmia
    c. Respiration
    d. Temperature

17. Which word means <u>wet</u>?
    a. Mildewed
    b. Moist
    c. Arid
    d. Temperate

18. Select the meaning of the underlined word. With her floppy hats and colorful dresses, she was often considered quite <u>eccentric</u>.
    a. Happy
    b. Frightening
    c. Odd
    d. Unhappy

19. Select the correct word order.
    a. The cat was hungry, so I fed it.
    b. I fed it so the cat was hungry
    c. The cat fed it, so was hungry.
    d. I fed the cat, so I was hungry.

20. Select the meaning of the underlined word. People with a suppressed immune system are <u>vulnerable</u> to infection.
    a. Safe
    b. Susceptible
    c. Powerful
    d. Weak

21. Select the word or phrase that is grammatically correct. _____ your homework last night or this morning?
    a. Will you finish
    b. Did you finish
    c. Have you finished
    d. Would you finish

22. Select the meaning of the underlined word. The company is well-known for its <u>sound</u> business practices.
    a. Audible
    b. Sensible
    c. Bad
    d. Excellent

23. Which word means <u>old</u>?
    a. Juvenile
    b. Pediatric
    c. Obstetric
    d. Geriatric

24. Which word that means <u>dead</u> best fits this sentence? She worked at the newspapers, writing obituaries for the _____.
    a. Murdered
    b. Extinct
    c. Lifeless
    d. Deceased

25. Select the correct word order.
    a. I bought a present for him.
    b. I for him bought a present.
    c. A present for him I bought.
    d. For him I bought a present.

26. Which word is a synonym for <u>beautiful</u>?
    a. Banal
    b. Comely
    c. Homely
    d. Tedious

27. Select the correct word order.
    a. The trains offered a high-speed transportation alternative.
    b. A high-speed transportation alternative offered the trains.
    c. The trains alternative high-speed transportation offered.
    d. The trains a high-speed transportation alternative offered.

28. Which word means <u>lacking sensation</u>?
    a. Sensate
    b. Numb
    c. Sensational
    d. Tingling

29. Which word is not spelled correctly?
    a. Insicion
    b. Surgical
    c. Orthopedic
    d. Podiatrist

30. Which word is a synonym for <u>dull</u>?
    a. Lustrous
    b. Vivacious
    c. Wearisome
    d. Underprivileged

31. Select the word or phrase that is grammatically correct. I _____ the patient to his room, checked his vitals and started an I.V.
    a. Helped
    b. Help
    c. Will help
    d. Did help

32. Which word is not spelled correctly?
    a. Weight
    b. Height
    c. Cardiac
    d. Resperatory

33. Which word is not spelled correctly?
    a. Coul'dnt
    b. You're
    c. It's
    d. Won't

34. Which word is a synonym for <u>tasteless</u>?
    a. Pulchritude
    b. Bland
    c. Vacuous
    d. Impassive

35. Select the word or phrase that is grammatically correct. I went ___ the store to buy milk and eggs.
    a. For
    b. From
    c. Up
    d. To

36. Which word is not spelled correctly?
    a. Affect
    b. Effect
    c. Affective
    d. Effortless

37. Which word means help?
    a. Hinder
    b. Assist
    c. Mediate
    d. Abrogate

38. Select the word or phrase that is grammatically correct. Last month, the patient _____ of chest pains.
    a. Complained
    b. To complain
    c. Complains
    d. Will complain

39. What is the best description of the underlined part of the sentence? I went to school early for basketball practice.
    a. Adjective
    b. Preposition
    c. Prepositional phrase
    d. Adverb

40. Select the meaning of the underlined word. They were an affectionate family, frequently playing and laughing together.
    a. Loving
    b. Unhappy
    c. Dysfunctional
    d. Tired

41. Select the meaning of the underlined word. He was driven, finishing his college degree in three years.
    a. Lazy
    b. Ambitious
    c. Bored
    d. Dumb

42. Select the meaning of the underlined word. His responses and personality were <u>brusque</u>.
    a. Cheerful
    b. Slow
    c. Curt
    d. Angry

43. Select the meaning of the underlined word. The test caused him to feel <u>apprehensive</u>.
    a. Nervous
    b. Terrified
    c. Excited
    d. Elated

44. Select the meaning of the underlined word. She was <u>deferential</u> to her supervisors.
    a. Disrespectful
    b. Respectful
    c. Rude
    d. Pleasant

45. Select the meaning of the underlined word. She was <u>conscientious</u> about patient care.
    a. Careless
    b. Sloppy
    c. Careful
    d. Slow

46. Select the meaning of the underlined word. You should be <u>amicable</u> and professional when dealing with the families of your patients.
    a. Cold
    b. Friendly
    c. Unfriendly
    d. Funny

47. Select the meaning of the underlined word. Social workers will investigate <u>alleged</u> child abuse.
    a. Proven
    b. False
    c. Unproven
    d. Terrible

48. Select the meaning of the underlined word. At work, your jewelry should be small and <u>inconspicuous.</u>
    a. Noticeable
    b. Unremarkable
    c. Bold
    d. Boring

49. Select the meaning of the underlined word. Be careful not to <u>neglect</u> your record-keeping duties at work.
      a. Forget
      b. Ignore
      c. Overdo
      d. Incorporate

50. Select the meaning of the underlined word. Don't forget to give the patients <u>assessments</u> to fill out before their appointments.
      a. Questionnaires
      b. Examinations
      c. Records
      d. Measurements

<u>Vocabulary Practice Test #2 – ANSWER KEY</u>

1. A
2. D
3. D
4. B
5. B
6. D
7. B
8. A "Let go" is a euphemism for fired.
9. D Lisensed should be licensed.
10. A
11. C
12. D
13. A
14. B
15. C
16. C
17. B
18. C
19. A
20. B
21. B
22. B
23. D
24. D
25. A I bought a present for him is correct. I is the subject, bought the verb and a present the direct object.
26. B
27. A The trains offered a high-speed transportation alternative. The trains is the subject, offered the verb, and alternative the direct object. High-speed and transportation are adjectives describing the alternative.
28. B
29. A Insision should be incision.
30. C
31. A Helped is correct. The other verbs are all past tense.
32. D Resperatory should be respiratory.
33. A Coul'dnt should be couldn't.
34. B
35. D To the store is the correct response, as the other prepositions do not refer to going toward something.
36. C Affective should be effective.
37. B
38. A Complained, as the incident happened in the past.
39. C For is a preposition, so "for basketball practice" is a prepositional phrase.
40. A
41. B
42. C

43. A
44. B
45. C
46. B
47. C
48. B
49. B
50. A

BIOLOGY PRACTICE TEST #2

1. How many pairs of human chromosomes exist?
   A. 17
   B. 13
   C. 23
   D. 29

2. Animals engaging in a symbiotic relationship will do which of the following?
   A. Help each other survive
   B. Take one another's food
   C. Attack one another
   D. Eat each other

3. What organ system contains your skin?
   A. The respiratory system
   B. The epithelial system
   C. The lymphatic system
   D. The circulatory system

4. If a gene is expressed, then that means that:
   A. It is influencing a phenotype trait
   B. It is being copied into another set of DNA
   C. It will be passed on from mother to son
   D. The gene will produce some hormones

5. Which of the following structures is found in eukaryotes but not in prokaryotes?
   A. A cell wall
   B. Mitochondria
   C. A nuclear membrane
   D. Vacuoles

6. A mutation in DNA can be caused by all of the following except:
   A. Ultraviolet radiation
   B. Chemical exposure
   C. DNA replication error
   D. Exonic duplication

7. People who suffer from Type I diabetes are lacking function in which organ?
   A. Liver
   B. Pancreas
   C. Stomach
   D. Heart

8. One of the primary differences between fungi and plants is that:
   A. Fungi can produce their own food and plants cannot.
   B. Plants have chlorophyll and fungi do not.
   C. Fungi are able to grow without water and plants cannot.
   D. Fungi and plants have no major differences.

9. Which of the following organisms is capable of asexual reproduction?
   A. Squash plant
   B. Amoeba
   C. Salmon
   D. Koala bear

10. In our atmosphere, nitrogen is the most common element, and makes up approximately what percentage?
    A. 25%
    B. 51%
    C. 65%
    D. 78%

11. In the human body, which of the following is responsible for clotting blood?
    A. Platelets
    B. White blood cells
    C. Red blood cells
    D. Osteoplasts

12. In plants, the female reproductive structures reside in the pistil, whereas the male reproductive structures are in the:
    A. Stamen
    B. Anther
    C. Sepals
    D. Petals

13. In the human body, communication occurring from cell to cell can happen through the use of:
    A. Neurotransmitters
    B. Pili
    C. Flagella
    D. ATP

14. In the following list, which would be considered to be at the top of the food chain?
    A. Snake
    B. Mouse
    C. Hawk
    D. Tomato plant

15. Tundra, rainforest, and prairie are all examples of ecological classifications known as:
    A. Ecomes
    B. Partitions
    C. Biomes
    D. Communities

16. Which of the following species is not important in DNA transcription and translation?
    A. mRNA
    B. tRNA
    C. Ribosome
    D. All of the above are important

17. A researcher is trying to create some protein, and is trying to get a ribosome to read the DNA he has prepared. This will not work, because:
    A. Ribosomes can only read DNA if tRNA is present.
    B. Ribosomes can only read RNA, not DNA.
    C. The DNA is double stranded and not single stranded, which is required for a ribosome to use.
    D. This should work, and nothing is wrong.

18. Which phase of the cell cycle requires the most time?
    A. Metaphase
    B. Interphase
    C. Telokinesis
    D. Longisphase

19. A haploid cell that is used to reproduce in a sexually reproductive organism is called a:
    A. Blastocoel
    B. Gamete
    C. Zygote
    D. Barr body

20. Which of the following species would not use meiosis as a cell process?
    A. Elephant
    B. Oak tree
    C. Salmon
    D. E. coli

21. What is the backbone of a DNA molecule made of?
    A. Protein
    B. Lipid
    C. Sugar
    D. Phenol

22. In eukaryotes, DNA is typically found in the:
    A. Cytoplasm
    B. Nucleus
    C. Endoplasmic reticulum
    D. Cell membrane

23. Different organisms obtain their energy from different sources. For example, plants are autotrophs and create their own food, whereas most animals are heterotrophs, eating other organisms for energy. However, all of this energy is derived from:
    A. Kinetic energy
    B. Light energy
    C. Adenosine tri-phosphate
    D. Bond energy

24. In the diagram below, the cell could be best classified as a:

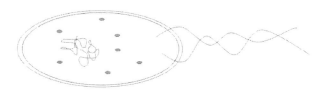

    A. Eukaryote
    B. Virus
    C. Blood cell
    D. Moneran

25. Which of the following statements regarding life on earth is *not* true?
    E. The major elements in living organisms are carbon, oxygen, nitrogen, and silicon.
    F. Many living creatures consume the remains of other organisms to acquire organic carbon.
    G. Trace elements, such as iron, potassium, or sulfur, are required by a majority of living organisms.
    H. Plants provide the major source of carbon for the kingdom Animalia.

Biology Practice Test #2 Answer Key

1. C
2. A
3. B
4. A
5. C
6. D
7. B
8. B
9. B
10. D
11. A
12. B
13. A
14. C
15. C
16. D
17. B
18. B
19. B
20. D
21. C
22. B
23. B
24. D
25. A

CHEMISTRY PRACTICE TEST #2

1. Perform the following calculation: $1.2 \times 10^2 + 7.8 \times 10^4$
   a) 7812
   b) 78120
   c) 781200
   d) 7812000

2. Sam has produced data from an experiment, and one of the values he reads out is 1.28000×10^3. What is not correct about this number?
   a) The number should be rounded to 1.3
   b) The number should have 2 more significant figures
   c) The number's zeroes on the end are not significant and should not be included
   d) This number is correct, and nothing is wrong

3. Convert a speed of 50 kilometers per hour into meters per second.
   a) 11.5 m/s
   b) 12.1 m/s
   c) 15.5 m/s
   d) 13.9 m/s

4. How many cubic centimeters (cm^3) are there in a cubic meter?
   a) 1×10^3
   b) 1×10^6
   c) 1×10^9
   d) 10,000

5. A standard light bulb uses about 60 watts, which is equivalent to 60 Joules per second (J/s). How many Btu's per second is it using?
   a) 0.034
   b) 3.5×10^{-3}
   c) 5.6×10^{-2}
   d) 0.00045

6. Absolute zero is the lowest temperature possible, and is represented by 0 K. What is this temperature in Celsius?
   a) -100 °C
   b) -193 °C
   c) -273 °C
   d) -373 °C

7. Room temperature in the United States is commonly referred to as 70 °F, which is approximately:
   a) 28 °C
   b) 529 °R
   c) 197 K
   d) None of the above

8. What is the reason for your answer to question **5**?
    g) This chemical reaction destroys matter.
    h) Matter is consumed by the flame.
    i) The mass of ash is less than the match it came from.
    j) The atoms are not destroyed, they are only rearranged.
    k) The match weighs less after burning.

9. An unsaturated solution:
    a) Hasn't dissolved as much solute as is theoretically possible.
    b) Has dissolved exactly as much solute as is theoretically possible.
    c) Is unstable because it has dissolved more solute than would be expected.
    d) None of the above.

10. If the pressure of water is kept below its triple point, and the temperature is increased, ice will:
    a) Turn to liquid
    b) Turn to gas
    c) Remain the same
    d) Become more crystalline

11. Which of the following is true regarding molecules in water vapor at 100 °C?
    a) They have less energy than liquid water at 100 °C
    b) They have more energy than liquid water at 100 °C
    c) They will condense into liquid if the pressure is reduced.
    d) There will be both liquid and vapor if the temperature is increased slightly.

12. A scientist has 1 mol of a sample of gas at 0°C and 1 atm of pressure. How much volume will it occupy?
    a) 18.5 liters
    b) 19.9 liters
    c) 22.4 liters
    d) 25.2 liters

13. A scientist has discovered what he thinks to be a new element! It has 45 protons and 52 neutrons. It is most likely:
    a) Palladium
    b) Silver
    c) Rhodium
    d) Cobalt

14. How many protons does Strontium have?
    a) 15
    b) 30
    c) 38
    d) 42

15. Susan has discovered an odd atom. It has 15 protons and a whopping 20 neutrons. This electron is likely to be:
    a) Sulfur
    b) Radioactive
    c) Heavier than gold
    d) Stable

16. Which of the following pairs of elements are *not* likely to form a bond?
    a) Na & Cl
    b) B & S
    c) Ca & O
    d) Fe & I

17. Which of the following is a true statement about the periodic table?
    a) The size of elements increases from right to left
    b) The electron shell size increases from top to bottom
    c) The electronegativity increases from top to bottom
       The radioactivity of elements decreases from left to right

18. Which of the following produces a gas from a solid?
    a) Melting
    b) Plasmification
    c) Condensation
    d) Sublimation

19. A student isolates a substance, and succeeds in purifying it. She then puts it into the lab refrigerator, at 4 °C. When she comes back the next day, she notices that it has solidified! Which of the following statements should be true about the substance?
    a) It has a melting point below 4 °C
    b) It has a boiling point less than that of water
    c) It has a freezing point higher than that of water
    d) It has a vaporization point at around 90 °C

20. What are the products of the following reaction?

$$NaOH + HCl \rightarrow ?$$

    a) Dihydrogen monoxide and sodium chloride
    b) Sodium hydride and chlorohydroxide
    c) Hydrochloride and sodium monohydroxide
    d) Sodium chloride and sodium hydroxide

21. In the following chemical reaction, what is the correct stoichiometric coefficient for silicon dioxide?

$$4Si + 2O_2 \rightarrow Si + SiO_2$$

   a) 1
   b) 2
   c) 3
   d) 4

22. In the following reaction, which species is the reducing agent?
   $3H_2S + 2HNO_3 \rightarrow 3S + 2NO + 4H_2O$

   a) Sulfur
   b) Nitrate
   c) Hydrogen
   d) Nitrogen

23. In the same reaction above, which species is being reduced?
   a) Sulfur
   b) Nitrogen
   c) Hydrogen
   d) Water

24. An oxidation/reduction reaction will not usually occur between lithium and sodium. What is a possible reason for this?
   a) They are both negatively charged alkali metals
   b) Their electronegativity values are too close
   c) They are transition metals, which do not participate in redox reactions
   d) Their electron shells do not have enough electrons

25. In the reactant potassium nitrate (KNO_3), what is the oxidation state of nitrogen?
   a) +2
   b) +3
   c) +4
   d) +5

Chemistry Practice Test #2 Answer Key

1. B
2. C
3. D
4. B
5. C
6. C
7. B
8. D
9. A
10. B
11. B
12. C
13. C
14. C
15. B
16. B
17. B
18. D
19. C
20. A
21. B
22. A
23. B
24. B
25. D

ANATOMY & PHYSIOLOGY
PRACTICE TEST #2

1. The conduction of air through the respiratory system follows which of the following paths?
   a) Pharynx, larynx, alveoli, trachea, bronchus, bronchioles.
   b) Alveoli, bronchioles, bronchus, trachea, larynx, pharynx.
   c) Pharynx, larynx, trachea, bronchus, bronchioles, alveoli.
   d) Bronchus, bronchioles, alveoli, pharynx, larynx, trachea.

2. The lungs are very efficient at gas exchange because they have a:
   a) High mass.
   b) Low volume.
   c) High surface-area-to-volume ratio.
   d) Low surface-area-to-volume ratio.

3. Fluid skeletal systems are _____.
   a) Hydrostatic.
   b) Hydrolic.
   c) Hydrophobic.
   d) Hydroskeleton.

4. The chief function of the colon is to:
   a) Absorb water from undigested waste.
   b) Produce sugars.
   c) Absorb protein from undigested waste.
   d) Produce carbohydrates.

5. Peristalsis is a process performed by which type of muscle tissue?
   a) Catabolic.
   b) Cardiac.
   c) Smooth.
   d) Skeletal.

6. Capillary beds occur between:
   a) Arteries and veins.
   b) Aortas and vena cavas.
   c) Arterioles and venules.
   d) Atria and ventricles.

7. Which of the following is **NOT** a function of the kidneys?
    a) Regulating pH (acidity) of blood.
    b) Regulating blood pressure.
    c) Assisting in the maintenance of homeostasis.
    d) Regulating hormone release.

8. Which of the following is a part of the CNS?
    a) Autonomic nerves.
    b) Sympathetic nerves.
    c) Peripheral nerves.
    d) Spinal cord nerves.

9. Which of the following is NOT true about irritability?
    a) Plants do not experience irritability.
    b) Activates neurons in the brain.
    c) Requires axons in animals.
    d) Neurons act upon muscles.

10. The most important gland in the human body is:
    a) The pancreas.
    b) The pituitary.
    c) The ovaries.
    d) The thyroid.

11. _____ is the functional unit of the nervous system.
    a) The nephron
    b) The nucleus
    c) The neuron
    d) The neutrophil

12. What two protein molecules are needed for muscles to contract?
    a) Pepsin and insulin.
    b) Myosin and pepsin.
    c) Hemoglobin and insulin.
    d) Myosin and actin.

13. Food begins the digestive process in the:

    a) Esophagus.

    b) Stomach.

    c) Intestines.

    d) Mouth.

14. Spermatogenesis is a process that happens in:

    a) The prostate

    b) The testis

    c) The urethra

    d) None of the above

15. In female organs, the urethra empties:

    a) Outside the body

    b) In the labia minor

    c) In the labia major

    d) None of the above

16. Which of the urethral sphincters can we control?

    a) The internal urethral sphincter

    b) The external urethral sphincter

    c) All of the urethral sphincters

    d) None of the above

17. Where does digestion start?

    a) The stomach

    b) The small intestine

    c) The mouth

    d) None of the above

18. The large intestine:

    a) Absorbs water

    b) Digests food

    c) Moves the food from the esophagus to the small intestine

    d) None of the above

19. Where does integration happen?

    a) ANS

    b) CNS

    c) PNS

    d) None of the above

20. Which part of the PNS is responsible for the fight or flight reaction?
   a) The parasympathetic
   b) The sympathetic
   c) The ENS.
   d) None of the above

21. What is the name of a state of constant muscle contraction caused by rapid successive nerve signals?
   a) Tetanus
   b) Muscle tone
   c) Temporal summation
   d) None of the above

22. Which of the following can be found in abundance in a fatigues muscle?
   a) Glucose
   b) Lactic acid
   c) ATP
   d) None of the above

23. What is the name of the process that happens in the red bone marrow?
   a) Hematopoiesis
   b) Bone fusing
   c) Calcification
   d) None of the above

24. The vertebral column protects the:
   a) Brain
   b) Heart
   c) Spinal column
   d) None of the above

25. The tidal volume is the amount of air moved during:
   a) Deep breathing
   b) Shallow breathing
   c) Coughing
   d) None of the above

Anatomy & Physiology Practice Test #2 – ANSWER KEY

1. C
2. C
3. A
4. A
5. C
6. C
7. D
8. D
9. A
10. B
11. C
12. D
13. D
14. B
15. B
16. B
17. C
18. A
19. B
20. B
21. A
22. B
23. A
24. C
25. B

PHYSICS PRACTICE TEST #2

1. **Which of the following is not a correct unit for the amount of work done:**
   a) Joule
   b) Horsepower-hour
   c) Calorie
   d) Newton

2. **Observe the figure:**

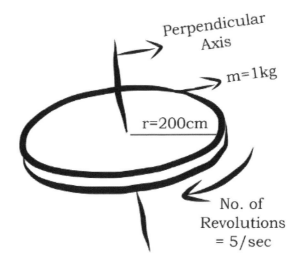

Perpendicular Axis

$m = 1kg$

$r = 200cm$

No. of Revolutions = 5/sec

   The kinetic energy of the disc is:
   a) $80 \, \pi^2 \, J$
   b) $100 \, \pi^2 \, J$
   c) $125 \, \pi^2 \, J$
   d) $144 \, \pi^2 \, J$

3. Consider the following figure of a rolling wheel on smooth horizontal surface:

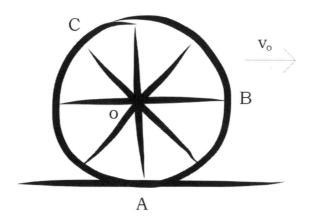

    Then,
    i.   Speed at the point **A** is 0
    ii.   Speed at point **B** & **C** = v_o
    iii.   Speed at point **B** > Speed at point **O**

    a) All the statements are true
    b) Only statement (i) & (ii) are true
    c) Only statement (i) & (iii) are true
    d) Only statement (ii) & (iii) are true

4. In the following figure, consider a block of mass m. What is the ratio of the force required, for a person to lift the block upwards with & without a pulley[BH11]? (Hint: Assume F=T)
    a) 2
    b) 1/3
    c) 3
    d) ½

5. A block of mass 3kg lies on a horizontal surface with μ = 0.7, select the force closest to what is required to just move the block:
    a) 15N
    b) 21N
    c) 18N
    d) 24N

6. P is a block of mass 5kg. At point Q, a block of mass 3kg was attached to just slide the block P.

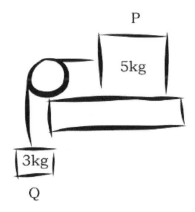

   If no displacement occurs, the coefficient of friction between the block P and the horizontal surface is:
   a) 0.5
   b) 0.6
   c) 0.7
   d) 0.8

7. A ball is thrown in the air, after few seconds, it returns back to the earth. What can be its likely cause?
   a) Earth's gravitational field pulls it back
   b) It's speed did not match the escape velocity of earth
   c) Neither of these is correct
   d) Both (a) and (b) are correct

8. The factor which distinguishes between a scalar and a vector quantity is:
   a) Magnitude
   b) Direction
   c) Both (a) & (b)
   d) Neither (a) nor (b)

9. An athlete couldn't stop himself immediately after crossing the finish line. He was explained why this was happening by Newton's:
   a) 1st law of motion
   b) 2nd law of motion
   c) 3rd law of motion
   d) Law of Universal Gravitation

10. How is the weight of a person in an elevator affected if the elevator accelerates upwards, accelerates downwards and is at at rest?
   a) Increases, Decreases, Remains Constant
   b) Decreases, Remains Constant, Increases
   c) Remains Constant, Increases, Decreases
   d) Decreases, Increases , Remains Constant

11. **In the above example of a lift, which of Newton's law is demonstrated?**
    a) 1st law of motion
    b) 2nd law of motion
    c) 3rd law of motion
    d) Law of Universal Gravitation

12. **The threads of a screw work on the principle of another type of simple machine, which is:**
    a) Lever
    b) Inclined plane
    c) Wedge
    d) None of the above

13. **The shaft of the screw penetrates wood through the principle of yet another simple machine, which is:**
    a) Inclined plane
    b) Lever
    c) Wedge
    d) None of the above

14. **The following objects are an example of which order of the lever:**
    Forceps, Scissors, Fishing Rod, Bottle Opener
    a) 3rd, 2nd, 3rd, 1st
    b) 2nd, 3rd, 1st, 3rd
    c) 3rd, 1st, 3rd, 2nd
    d) 1st, 3rd, 2nd, 3rd

15. **A mechanic observes that he is able to lift the car by 2cm if he moves down the lever by 30cm. if he is applying a force of 20N to the lever, the force applied by the lever on the car is:**
    a) 250N
    b) 300N
    c) 350N
    d) 400N

16. **Angular momentum of a body doesn't change if:**
    a) External torque is not applied
    b) External torque is applied in CW Direction
    c) External torque is applied in CCW Direction
    d) External torque has no effect on the angular momentum of the body

Physics Practice Test #2 – ANSWER KEY

1. **Ans. (d)**
   Work is equal to the force multiplied by the displacement in the direction of the force. Newton is a unit of measurement for force, so the correct unit for amount of work is Nm, which is equal to Joule.

2. **Ans. (b)**
   m = 1kg; r = 200cm = 2m; n = 5; w = 2pin = 2pi5 = 10pi K.E. = 1/2Iw2 = 1/2*1/2*mr2w2 = 1/2*1/2*1*22*(10pi)2

3. **Ans. (c)**
   In case of rolling motion without slipping, the point touching the ground is always instantaneously at zero velocity. Hence velocity of point A is 0.
   The centre of the wheel always remains at a constant linear velocity in such type of motion. Hence the speed at point O which is the centre of the wheel is v_o.

4. **Ans. (d)**
   With pulley: F + T[BH12] = mg
   2F = mg
   Fwp = mg/2
   Without pulley: Fwop = mg
   Fwp/Fwop = mg/2/mg = ½

5. **Ans. (b)**
   Vertical forces are in equilibrium:
   uR => umg
   Therefore, F = uR = umg = 0.7*3*9.8 = 20.58N

6. **Ans. (b)**
   F = T
   umg = 3g
   u = 3/m = 3/5 = 0.6

7. **Ans. (d)**
   Both options are correct.

8. **Ans. (b)**
   A scalar quantity has only magnitude, whereas a vector quantity has magnitude as well as direction.

9. **Ans. (a)**
   Remember inertia of motion. An object in motion stays in motion and an object at rest stays at rest unless acted on by an external force.

10. Ans. (a)

When the lift is accelerating upwards, the weight of a person (called apparent weight) becomes: $F = mg + ma$

When the lift is accelerating downwards, the weight of a person becomes: $F = mg - ma$

When the lift is at rest, the weight of a person remains constant i.e. $F = mg$

11. Ans. (c)

To every action there is an equal and opposite reaction i.e. Newton's 3rd law.[BH13]

12. Ans. (b)

Threads of a screw can also be viewed as an inclined plane.

13. Ans. (c)

The shaft of the screw has a pointed end which works on the principle of a wedge.

14. Ans. (c)

Forceps and fishing rod are an example of 3rd order lever with effort being applied between load and fulcrum.

Scissors are an example of 1st order lever with fulcrum at the centre.

Bottle opener is an example of 2nd order lever with load being between fulcrum and effort arm.

15. Ans. (b)

$d_E*F_E = d_R*F_R$

$30*20 = 2*x$

$x = 300N$

16. Ans. (a)

Angular momentum is the product of Moment of Inertia and Angular velocity and is given by $L = I\omega$

When no external torque is applied, the angular velocity is 0 which is given by $\omega = 2\pi n$ where n is the number of revolutions a body has due to external torque applied. Hence, angular momentum of a body does not change if external torque is not applied.

Made in the USA
Middletown, DE
10 February 2015